THE

GOUT COOKBOOK

&

DIET GUIDE

-----------------~-----------------

85 Healthy Homemade & Low Purine Recipes for People with Gout Disease

-----------------~-----------------

ALSO INCLUDES: A COMPREHENSIVE DIET AND CURE GUIDE FOR GOUT

BY

MONIKA SHAH

COPYRIGHT © 2015

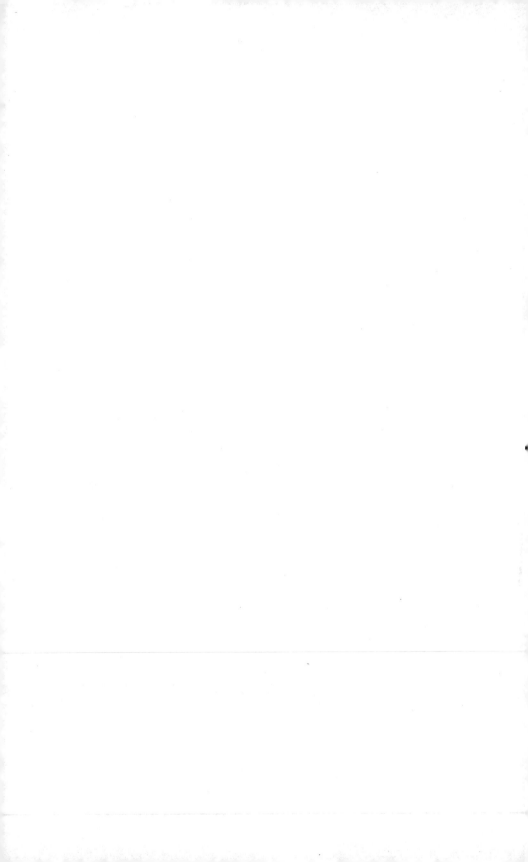

A Message for Readers!

Heal & Cure Your Gout Disease with the Right Diet & Management

This book has been specifically designed and written for people who have been suffering with Gout and seriously strive to heal and cure it with the help of a healthy, low purine and effective homemade diet. Apart from taking medications prescribed by the doctor, it is extremely important to eat the right and low purine diet to maintain the right purine levels in the body to help reduce Gout attacks.

Let's take a closer look on what this book has to offer:

- **The Gout Disease Cookbook:** The cookbook has 85 healthy homemade & low purine recipes which are designed especially for people with Gout. The recipes in the book have been designed using very simple ingredients that people use in their kitchen every day or can find in the grocery stores very easily. These recipes are further categorized into **Breakfast, Lunch, Dinner, Salads, Dips, Snacks, Drinks** and **Desserts**.

  The whole purpose of these recipes is to make sure that the person with Gout enjoys life without compromising the taste of the real food. Each recipe in this book has easy to find ingredients and steps with accurate serving sizes. You will find recipes which can be eaten daily or on occasions without even compromising with health a bit.

- **The Gout Disease Diet Guide:** The primary focus of this part of the book is to guide you on what kind of diet and foods you must eat if you have Gout. This section comes with a list of 224 foods along with their purine levels. These foods have been further categorized into three different lists, **Foods highest in Purine, Foods Moderately High in Purine** and **Foods Lowest in Purine**. These organized lists will help you identify the foods that you should be eating and avoiding.

- **The Gout Prevention & Cure Guide:** This part of the book not only helps you with the preventive measures but also to heal and cure gout using various tested and proven natural home-based remedies, therapies, oil treatments and other methods. This dedicated part of the book will help you with an effective management of Gout disease and live pain free.

CONTENTS

Copyright Notes & Disclaimer

No part of this Book can be reproduced in any form or by any means including print, electronic, scanning or photocopying unless prior permission is granted by the author. This e-book is licensed for your personal use only and may not be re-sold or given away to other people. If you would like to share this book with other person, please purchase an additional copy for each recipient.

All ideas, suggestions and guidelines mentioned here are written for informative purposes. While the author has taken every possible step to ensure the accuracy, all readers are advised to follow information at their own risk. The author cannot be held responsible for personal and/or commercial damages in case of misinterpreting any part of this book.

All attempts have been made by the author to provide factual and accurate content. No responsibility will be taken by the author for any damages caused by misuse of the content described in this book. The content of this book has been derived from various sources. Please consult a licensed professional before attempting any techniques outlined in this book.

This Page Has Been Left Blank Intentionally.

PART A –UNDERSTANDING GOUT

This Page Has Been Left Blank Intentionally.

Chapter 1

Understanding Gout Disease and

Its Symptoms

Many centuries ago, Gout was also called a rich man's disease or a king's disease. It was the luxuries afforded by the wealthy, eating meat and consuming alcohol that caused its flare up and hence the nickname. However, today it is a commoner's condition. In fact, so much so that between 3 and 6 million Americans are reportedly affected by it.

You may not believe this but gout goes all the way back to 2640 BC, when it was first identified by the Ancient Egyptians. At the turn of 5th Century BC, Hippocrates was the first iconic Greek physician to talk about gout as an "un-walkable disease". He developed the connection between lifestyle habits and the development of condition in the people at that time.

Gout is not a "status" condition anymore. It is more communal than it should be! This form of inflammatory arthritis is very painful and can cause excruciating pain, swelling of the joints, and redness in the affected area. If you have gout problem, chances are it is in the big toe zone; but, it is not just limited to this area. Other commonly affected parts of the body include other joints in the foot, elbow, wrist and the fingertips.

There are many triggers that can cause an episode of gout or the symptoms to occur without so much as a warning. There are people who report a flare up in the middle of the night too! Sometimes the pain lasts for days and sometimes it can go up to weeks, with first two days being the worst. Even though there is still a lot of clarity required on why gout happens in the first place, there are lot of well-established treatments and diagnosis for this condition.

Gout may be an old disease, stemming centuries back. However, it is an imminent public health concern even today. There are more and more people suffering from this painful condition every day. Gout is not just a bearer of arthritis but it also increases the risk of cardiovascular and metabolic disease amongst the people affected by it. Despite its popularity, there is still an acute lack of awareness amongst the people.

This book will walk you through the nuances of the disease because you need to know why your ankle is hurting the way it does. This book will serve as a guide to help you prevent this condition. However, if you already have it, it will help you understand what you are up against!

Anytime your body has inexplicable pain, don't wait for it to get worse. Take heed of the warning signs and check with your GP immediately.

What is Gout?

Resulting from the uric acid crystals build-up in the joint, gout can be called a collection of microscopic crystals in the joint's soft tissue that causes agonizing pain, swelling, redness and warmth.

The uric-acid crystals build-up begins in the body with a chemical compound called purines that are found in many foods. Uric acid is produced by the body when it metabolizes the purines which are then transferred into the bloodstream. This uric acid then exits the system with the help of kidney by excretion via urine or stool. However, when there is too much uric acid in the bloodstream, known as hyperuricemia, it leads to the formation of crystals that collect in the joints and cause gout.

This inability to adequately excrete the uric acid from the body is the leading cause of gout in people. Gout causes bursts of pain and swelling in more than one joint. For quick relief one can pop a painkiller to subside the pain but it is not a permanent solution. You need to change your lifestyle if you want more permanent relief from the problem. If you are overweight, consider losing weight, consume a healthy diet, and avoid drinking too much alcohol or soft drinks that have been artificially sweetened. You can prevent the gout attack by consuming vitamin c supplements every day.

If left untreated, a gout episode normally subsides on its own within a day or two. But if the problem recurs, it can be called a case of chronic gout that can lead to permanent damage to the joint over a period of time. This is the reason why it is important to diagnose and treat the problem at the first instance possible. The longer you wait, the higher you risk doing greater damage.

This is a very complex form of arthritis that is identified by the sudden bursts of pain that can be very severe. However, thankfully for those inflicted, gout is not only treatable but is also fully preventable by taking corrective measures for reducing the risk of developing this painful condition.

Is Gout Common?

Sadly, gout is more common than it should be. It affects 1 in 200 adults and men are more affected by gout than women. The first instance of gout normally happens as you approach the middle age. However, it may also happen to younger people too. If it runs in your family, your chances of developing gout become higher.

Who Gets It?

Millions of people are suffering from gout all over the world. Here is the type of people who are likely to get it:

- Men over the age of 40-years
- Women who have undergone menopause
- Obese people
- People who drink too much alcohol
- People on certain medication

Symptoms

Gout is a strange condition. It just sneaks up on you, out of nowhere! One night you may be sleeping peacefully when suddenly you get a gout attack, that too without a warning. Here are some signs that suggest you should talk to your GP about gout:

- **Intense pain in the joints:** This is the biggest sign of gout. When the large joint of your big toe pains inexplicably, perhaps it is time you get the tests done. It does not only impact the big toe region but also other parts of the body such as knees, feet, ankles and wrists. The pain in these areas is very severe within the first 12 hours after it begins.

- **Discomfort in the ligaments:** After the initial pain subsides, you may experience joint discomfort that can take a few days or even a week or more to pass completely. The attack later may last for longer period of time, while affecting more joints.

- **Redness and inflammation:** The parts of the body that are inflicted with gout will become tender, swollen, warm and red. You will notice this mainly in the joints area.

- **Limited mobility**: As gout occurs and further progresses, the mobility of your joints may be affected.

Time to See a Doctor

If you have been experiencing intense pain in your joints, then you need to call your doctor right now. If gout is left untreated, it can lead to joint damage or worsen the condition. If you experience hot and inflamed joint coupled with fever, it may be a sign of infection. This would be the time when you seek immediate medical attention.

This Page Has Been Left Blank Intentionally.

Chapter 2

How Gout Disease Develops

Once called the disease of the rich and famous, it was caused by eating too much food and drinking too much wine. Even though unhealthy eating and excessive drinking may contribute to the development of this disease, it will not be correct to call them the main reasons of the disorder.

Gout, as we discussed before, happens when the urate crystals accumulate in your joint. This causes serious inflammation and intense pain, also known as gout attack. The uric crystals form in the body when you have high levels of uric acid in your bloodstream.

The Uric Acid Build Up

In a normal healthy body, there is always a fine balance between the amount of uric acid that your body makes and the amount that you pass in the form of feces and urine. This keeps the uric acid levels in your body under control. However, in people that are suffering from gout, their kidneys do not release the fair amount of uric acid that leads to a rise in blood levels. Even though their kidneys work perfectly fine, these people are called the under-excreters of uric acid.

In most people, this build-up can happen due to one or combination of the many reasons mentioned below:

- Too much alcohol consumption leads to uric acid build up.
- When your body has vitamin C deficiency in your diet.
- Did you know that two drinks of sugar-sweetened soft drink can increase your risk of gout by 85%? Fructose causes uric acid build up in the body which is the main cause of gout.
- There are many foods that raise the uric acid levels in your body, usually higher than normal. Foods like herring, sardines, mussels and yeast extracts often tip the balance towards uric acid buildup. Consuming healthy diet of balanced nutrition keeps the levels in check.
- Some medicines may increase the uric acid levels in the body, such as chemotherapy, aspirin etc.
- When the cells in your body has rapid turnover, it leads to the production of uric acid even more. For example, psoriasis is one of the conditions that can lead to gout.

There are also other conditions that increase the risk of gout amongst people. These include:

- High blood pressure
- Diabetes mellitus
- Obesity
- Kidney failure
- Vascular conditions
- Bone marrow disorders
- Lipid conditions

Factors That Lead To Gout

When your body makes high levels of uric acid in your body, you become a potential candidate of gout. Factors that amplify the production of uric acid in your body include:

- **Unhealthy diet:** Consuming a diet that has high contents of meat and sea food can result in disturbing the uric acid balance in your body. Fructose present in most of the beverages or sweetened drinks promotes high uric acid levels that increase your risk of gout. Another most common aspect of gout is consumption of alcohol, especially beer.

- **Obesity:** When you are overweight, your body produces high levels of uric acid and your kidneys have a hard time in eliminating that uric acid from your body. As a result, you become more susceptible to the risk of gout. Additionally, high levels of body fat also lead to a rapid increase in systemic inflammation levels due to production of inflammatory cytokines made by the fat cells.

- **Pre-medical conditions:** There are certain conditions such as diabetes, kidney/heart diseases and metabolic syndrome that will most certainly culminate into gout at some point.

- **Medications:** The medicines that treat hypertension make you more vulnerable to gout. Even low-dose aspirin has been known to increase the uric acid levels in the body. If you ever underwent an organ transport, the anti-rejection drugs too can develop gout as a side effect.

- **Genetic:** If there is anyone in your family who has a history of gout, chances are you will develop it too!

- **Age and sex:** Gout most likely occurs in men because women have lower uric acid levels in the body. However, after menopause, women's body too makes almost the same amount of uric acid. Men can develop gout anytime between 30 and 50 years of age, while women become more susceptible to gout only after menopause.

- **Recent surgery or trauma:** If you have undergone surgery recently or have experienced trauma, you are likely to be exposed to the risk of developing gout.

Chapter 3

The Gout Disease Diagnosis

One of the most reliable methods of detecting the development of gout is by checking for uric acid crystals in the joint fluids. These fluids are obtained from the inflamed joint to check for gout. This fluid, extracted by the physicians, is then studied under the microscope to conclude the presence of uric crystals.

The Importance of Diagnosis

There are times when hot and stiff joints are caused by inflammatory arthritis that can also include gout. However, these symptoms may not always mean that it is gout. This is the reason it is important for the patient to undergo complete diagnosis and get suitable treatment for the condition. Gout is a terminal disease with a lifelong damage potential. This is why its diagnosis is absolutely necessary.

The Crystals

So you have been experiencing symptoms of gout and think it would be a good idea to get the tests done? The first thing that will make up your diagnosis is your history. Right from your age to weight, family history, sex and diet are considered contributing factors for gout. Sometimes even medications administered for cardiovascular and kidney problems too may cause development of gout.

The most accurate determinant of gout is the presence of uric acid crystals. If you can manage to visit your doctor during a gout attack, you will be able to ensure a precise diagnosis. The fluid is examined under a special microscope with filters that reveal the presence of crystals, if any.

The liquid is drained from the inflamed area in a short procedure that lasts for about 30 seconds to a minute. Although it can be slightly painful, doctors normally numb the area before they extract the fluid. Sometimes, crystals may not be visible in the fluid sample, however, that doesn't rule out the possibility of gout altogether. Further diagnosis may be required to determine the presence of gout, or its absence, for that matter.

Many people ask their doctors that why do they have to go through the painful process of fluid extraction and why can't a simple blood test do? This is because when you are experiencing a gout attack, it is not unheard of for the uric acid levels to be normal in blood. It is also possible to check the uric levels in urine sample but nothing detects it better than the inflamed joint fluid.

Other Signs and Symptoms

Other than the invasive process, there are physical signs too that can last longer than the acute gout period. One of the most common telltale signs is tophi, a thick deposit of uric crystals underneath the skin.

When your body shows signs of kidney stones and tophi, it means that the gout has been present for a number of years and the damage can be seen on the X-ray. The longer you wait for the treatment, the higher is the possibility of a kidney or joint damage. If you have an uncontrollable pain in your big toe, call your doctor immediately.

Here are some tests that will help determine the presence of gout.

- **Joint fluid test:** Your doctor draws out fluid from the affected area and examines under a microscope to look for uric crystals.

- **Dual energy CT scan:** Even if your joint is not really inflamed, this technique can still detect the presence of urate crystals. However, this test can be highly expensive, hence, is not used widely.

- **Ultrasound:** Musculoskeletal ultrasound helps determine presence of tophus or uric crystals in a joint.

- **X-ray imaging:** Joint x-rays are done to rule out other reasons that are causing the inflammation.

- **Blood test:** Sometimes they conduct a blood test to test the level of uric acid and creatinine present in your blood stream.

Since blood tests are not considered very reliable, it is better to go for other tests. Some people may have high uric acid levels but no gout and some may have normal uric acid but experience other symptoms of gout.

This Page Has Been Left Blank Intentionally.

Chapter 4

The Risks Associated with Gout

One of the most common, yet dangerously prevalent beliefs is that gout is a nonthreatening condition. According to them, even though it may cause a lot of pain, it doesn't lead to any real damage. However, this is a wrong belief because gout, if left undetected or untreated, can be very dangerous.

The Damage Done

Gout, as we discussed before, is an immune response of uric crystal formation in the joints. It is this immune response that is responsible for causing the pain as a result of inflammation in the joint. This inflammation can also cause permanent damage to the joint if the gout is not managed properly. Over the years, this damage can add up and become a source of constant pain in the joints, inhibiting its mobility. After a while, the joint will become stiff and unmovable and ultimately cause its complete immobilization.

Even though this may be extreme and not happen in every reported gout case but unmanaged gout condition can be very serious if left to its own devices. If your attacks occur occasionally, it will take longer for the gout to culminate into a permanent damage. However, if your gout attacks happen less frequently then it may never accumulate to a point where it causes any long term damage.

The other prevailing threat of untreated gout is tophus. This collection of uric acid crystals that form in your body is also an ever-present threat. Tophus usually forms around your joints but they are not restricted to this area. If untreated, tophus can become huge and permanently disfigure your hands, feet, knees and elbows. The most dangerous aspect of tophus is that they can also cause the skin above them to rupture, resulting in uric acid crystals to discharge from your body and cause infection.

The only way you can avoid this problem is by controlling the levels of uric acid in your body. If the uric levels are maintained below 6.8mg/dL, they will not be able to crystalize. The best way to stop tophus from forming is by lowering the uric acid levels.

The Hyperuricemia

As if tophus wasn't enough that you are also exposed to the dangers of hyperuricemia which has been established as the underlying cause of gout and a precursor to many diseases such as high blood pressure, kidney disease, liver disease, diabetes and obesity. What's worse? Research shows that by lowering your uric acids levels do not make a significant difference to reducing your risks of developing these diseases.

Hyperuricemia means that you have high levels of uric acid all over your body and not just your blood or joints. This means that even though you may have recommended levels of uric acid in your bloodstream, there may still be areas in your body that have high concentrations that are forming the crystals responsible for inflammation, even if they are not directly causing any gout attacks.

Apart from the inherent risk of gout itself, people with gout are exposed to other more severe conditions too, such as:

- **Kidney stones:** Sometimes the crystals accumulate in the urinary tract of people causing the risk of kidney stones.

- **Advanced gout:** When the gout is left untreated, it often causes the urate crystal deposits under the skin called tophi. It can develop on your hands, elbows, feet, fingers or Achilles tendons as well as the back of your ankles. Although they are not really painful as such, they do become tender when inflamed during gout attacks.

- **Recurrent gout:** While some people may never have to face the signs or symptoms of gout, there are others that experience gout many times during a year. These are the people that are suffering from recurrent attacks. Medication may help, but if left untreated, it can cause complete damage to the joint.

This Page Has Been Left Blank Intentionally.

PART B - THE DIET GUIDE &
COOKBOOK FOR GOUT

This Page Has Been Left Blank Intentionally.

Chapter 5

Diet Guidelines for Gout Disease

If you are a candidate for gout, what you eat or don't eat can play elemental role in triggering the condition in your body. Gout generally attacks the big toe region but can be experienced in other parts of the body too. Obese people and men are at a great risk. So if you are susceptible to gout, are a man or obese then you must certainly avoid these foods if you want to prevent gout and its flare up.

Foods to Exclude

The following is a high level list of foods that are considered high in purine levels and must not be consumed by people with Gout. For a complete and detailed list of foods with their purine levels, please refer to chapter 7.

- **Scallops:** When you are experiencing flare ups, say no to seafood for your own good. Animal foods are rich sources of purines that your body breaks into uric acid. If your gout has temporarily subsided, you may have the freedom to allow a little slip here and there, but it is still a good idea to maintain the seafood intake to a minimum of 4-6 ounces every day.

- **Herring:** Even though there are some sea-foods you can still enjoy, there are some options that shouldn't even be on your menu, especially when you have gout. Avoid eating herring, tuna, anchovies, to begin with. You can, however, consume shrimp, eel, lobster, hand and crab that are still considered safe.

- **Beer:** If you have gout, beer is your enemy. It not only increases the uric-acid levels but also makes it difficult for your body to clear it out from your system. Although it is better to eliminate alcohol altogether, if you must drink, let it be wine instead. Heavy drinking is bad for anyone and more so with people suffering from gout. During a flare, refrain from drinking alcohol completely.

- **Red meat:** One should always keep in mind that white meat is better than the red one and it is okay to eat meat every once in a while. It is better to occasionally indulge in beef or pork rather than lamb or turkey.

- **Turkey:** Turkey has high purine content and is best avoided. It is better to consume chicken or duck with leg meat than breast with skin.

- **Sugary beverages:** Avoid any drinks that are highly sweetened with fructose laden corn syrup such as "fruit" drinks. Drinking these beverages is the quickest way to gain weight and the sweeteners present in the drink will stimulate your body to create more uric acid. According to a recent study, men who consumed too much fructose were more exposed to the risk of developing gout.

- **Organ Meats:** Foods such as liver, kidneys etc. are laden with purines and are a strict no-no if you do not want to ever develop gout.

Foods to Include

Do you feel like all your food options have suddenly been eliminated? Don't! Because there are several foods out there that can prevent occurrence and recurrence of gout.

- **Stay hydrated:** When you supply your body with adequate liquids, it inhibits its ability to form the uric acid crystals that are responsible for gout. Water is the best source of fluid that can help pass uric acid through your body. You must drink at least 8 cups of water every day or up to 2 liters.

- **Eat foods rich in potassium:** Potassium helps passage of uric acid through your body. Foods like lima beans, cooked spinach, baked potatoes with skin and cantaloupes are high sources of potassium. If you are unable to include these in your diet, you can also take potassium supplements after consulting with your doctor.

- **Eat complex carbs:** People with gout are recommended to eat brown bread, fruits and vegetables in their daily diet.

- **Consume good quantities of Vitamin C:** Taking high quantities of vitamin C, as much as 1500-2000 mg per day can reduce the risk of gout, says study. Some people add a bit of lemon to their water each morning. However, you would require help of vitamin C supplements to reach this level.

- **Cherries are good:** This one is a folk remedy and is believed to treat gout while reducing your risk significantly. Cherries reduce the uric acid levels that in turn help prevent gout.

- **Milk and Dairy products:** Skimmed milk, low-fat yogurt and low-fat cottage cheese are great ways to prevent uric acid in blood. These foods provide your body with protein and are also low in purine content.

- **Tofu:** Tofu made using soybeans would be a better option and choice than meats. It is also a great option for people who are vegetarians or have stopped eating meats completely.

- **Celery:** Celery is a very popular and well known vegetable that helps reliving the symptoms of gout, rheumatism and arthritis.

Chapter 6

The Relation between Gout and Protein

Doctors recommend people who are gout-prone to avoid foods with high purine content, compounds that lead to the formation of uric acid. When these foods break down, they create excess uric acid which in most cases is flushed out of the body with the help of kidney. However, people with a risk of gout may find it hard to excrete the extra uric acid.

Even though your body may have high levels of uric acid, you may never experience a gout attack. However, sometimes your uric acid levels coupled with your hormones, genes and diet can trigger the symptoms. If you have gout risk due to genes or hormones, then high-protein diet can be dangerous for you.

Protein and Gout

People who are at risk of gout may be advised to follow a diet of low-proteins. Since high-protein contains loads of purines, it is better to avoid those foods altogether. It is the purines that crystalize in the joints and cause the gout attacks. Protein foods such as mackerel, goose, beef, organ meats and anchovies are some of the richest sources of purines.

Animal Protein in Moderation

Like said before, purine-rich foods increased the risk of gout amongst people. Protein from animal foods exposes you to a greater risk of gout than the plant protein. Only if the protein from animal is consumed in moderation is when you can offset the risk.

Plant Proteins are your Best Bet

Plant based foods are high protein foods but low in purines, except legumes, broccoli, bananas, apricots, peas and mushrooms. You can enjoy most of the fruits and vegetables without fearing the risk of gout attack. Best sources of plant based proteins are nuts, garbanzo beans, flaxseeds and sunflower seeds. The least purine content in ½ cup serving can be found in tofu, soybeans, red beans and pinto beans.

Safe consumption of Proteins

Even if you have never had gout in the past, eating too much protein may increase your risks of contracting one in the future. The belief that rich diet causes gout goes way back in history and does not take the current American diet into account.

Regardless of the threat, proteins are after all the building blocks of our body and are required for its healthy functioning. Here are some ways you can use to eat proteins safely in your diet without flaring up the gout.

- Do not eat more than 6 ounces of protein per day
- Only eat low-purine meats

Avoid organ meats like liver, kidneys, brains etc.

This Page Has Been Left Blank Intentionally.

Chapter 7

The Purine Levels: The A-Z List of 224 Foods with Purine Levels

People who suffer from Gout must know about the foods that are considered high, moderate and low in purine. This chapter will provide you an A-Z list of over 224 foods along with their purine content per 100 mg. This will help you in making right decisions while selecting your foods for Gout diet.

Foods Highest in Purine

The following is the list of foods that are considered highest in purines. The table shows the purine level in mg per 100g on average for each food listed below.

Foods	Total Purines in mg /100g (Average)
Fish, sardines in oil	480
Liver, Calf's	460
Mushroom, flat, edible Boletus, dried	488

Neck sweet bread, Calf's	1260
Ox liver	554
Ox spleen	444
Pig's heart	530
Pig's liver	515
Pig's lungs (lights)	434
Pig's spleen	516
Sheep's spleen	773
Sprat, smoked	804
Theobromine	2300
Yeast, Baker's	680
Yeast, Brewer's	1810

Foods Moderately High in Purine

The following is the list of foods that are considered moderately high in purines. The table shows the purine level in mg per 100g on average for each food listed below.

Foods	Total Purines in mg /100g (Average)
Bean, seed, white, dry	128
Bean, Soya, seed, dry	190
Beef, chuck	120
Beef, fillet	110
Beef, fore rib, entrecote	120
Beef, muscles only	133
Beef, roast beef, sirloin	110
Beef, shoulder	110
Black gram (mungo bean), seed, dry	222

Caviar (real)	144
Chicken (breast with skin)	175
Chicken (chicken for roasting), average	115
Chicken, boiling fowl, average	159
Chicken, leg with skin, without bone	110
Duck, average	138
Fish, Anchovy	239
Fish, Carp	160
Fish, Cod	109
Fish, Haddock	139
Fish, Halibut	178
Fish, Herring roe	190
Fish, Herring, Atlantic	210

Fish, Herring, Matje cured	219
Fish, Mackerel	145
Fish, Pike-perch	110
Fish, Redfish (ocean perch)	241
Fish, Saithe (coalfish)	163
Fish, salmon	170
Fish, sardine, pilchard	345
Fish, Sole	131
Fish, trout	297
Fish, Tuna	257
Fish, Tuna in oil	290
Goose	165
Grape, dried, raisin, sultana	107

Ham, cooked	131
Heart, Sheep's	241
Horse meat	200
Kidney, Calf's	218
Lamb (muscles only)	182
Lentil, seed, dry	127
Linseed	105
Liver, chicken	243
Lobster	118
Lungs, Calf's	147
Mussel	112
Ox heart	256
Ox kidney	269

Ox lungs (lights)	399
Ox tongue	160
Peas, chick (garbanzo), seed, dry	109
Pig's kidney	334
Pig's tongue	136
Pike	140
Poppy seed, seed, dry	170
Pork belly	100
Pork belly, raw, smoked dried	127
Pork chop with bone	145
Pork chuck	140
Pork fillet	150
Pork hip bone (hind leg)	120

Pork leg (hind leg)	160
Pork muscles only	166
Pork shoulder with skin (blade of shoulder)	150
Rabbit meat, average with bone	132
Rabbit/Hare (average)	105
Sausage "Jagdwurst"	112
Sausage salami, German	104
Sausage, liver (liverwurst)	165
Sausages, frying, from pork	101
Scallop	136
Shrimp, brown	147
Spleen, Calf's	343
Sunflower seed, dry	143

Turkey, young animal, average, with skin	150
Veal chop, cutlet with bone	140
Veal fillet	140
Veal knuckle with bone	150
Veal, leg of veal with bone	150
Veal, muscles only	172
Veal, neck with bone	150
Veal, shoulder	140
Venison back	105
Venison haunch (leg)	138

Foods Lowest in Purine

The following is the list of foods that are considered lowest in purines. The table shows the purine level in mg per 100g on average for each food listed below.

Foods	Total Purines in mg /100g (Average)
Almond, sweet	37
Apple	14
Apricot	73
Artichoke	78
Asparagus	23
Aubergine	21
Avocado	19
Bamboo Shoots	29
Banana	57

Barley without husk, whole grain	96
Bean sprouts, Soya	80
Beans, French (string beans, haricot)	37
Beans, French, dried	45
Beef, corned (German)	57
Beer, alcohol free	8.1
Beer, Pilsner lager beer, regular beer, German	13
Beer, real, light	14
Beet root	19
Bilberry, blueberry, huckleberry	22
Brain, Calf's	92
Bread, wheat (flour) or (white bread)	14
Broccoli	81

Brussels sprouts	69
Cabbage, red	32
Cabbage, savoy	37
Cabbage, white	22
Carrot	17
Cauliflower	51
Caviar substitute	18
Celeriac	30
Cheese, Brie	7.1
Cheese, Cheddar/Cheshire cheese, 50% fat content	6
Cheese, cottage	9.4
Cheese, edam, 30% fat content in dry matter	7.1
Cheese, edam, 40% fat content in dry matter	7.1

Cheese, edam, 45% fat content in dry matter	7.1
Cheese, Limburger, 20% fat content in dry matter	32
Cherry, Morello	17
Cherry, sweet	7.1
Chicory	12
Chinese leaves	21
Chives	67
Cocoa powder, oil partially removed, not including	71
Corn, sweet	52
Fish, Crayfish	60
Cress	28
Crispbread	60
Cucumber	7.3

Currant, red	17
Date, dried	35
Elderberry, black	33
Endive	17
Fennel leaves	14
Fig (dried)	64
Fish, eel (smoked)	78
Frankfurter sausages	89
Gooseberry	16
Grape	27
Grass, Viper's (black salsify)	71
Kale	48
Kiwi fruit (Chinese gooseberry, strawberry peach	19

Kohlrabi	25
Leek	74
Lettuce	13
Lettuce, Lamb's	38
Meat, luncheon	70
Melon, Cantelope	33
Millet, shucked corn	62
Morel	30
Mushroom	58
Mushroom, flat, edible Boletus, cep	92
Mushrooms, canned, solid and liquid	29
Mushrooms, Chanterelle	17
Mushrooms, Chanterelles, canned, solids & liquid	17

Nuts, Brazil	23
Nuts, hazelnut (cobnut)	37
Nuts, peanut	79
Oats, without husk, whole grain	94
Olive, green, marinated	29
Onion	13
Orange	19
Ox brain	75
Oyster	90
Oyster, mushroom	50
Parsley, leaf	57
Pasta made with egg (noodles, macaroni, spagh	40
Pea, pod and seed, green	84

Pea, seed, dry	95
Peach	21
Pear	12
Peppers, green	55
Pig's brain	83
Pineapple	19
Plaice	93
Plum	24
Plum, dried	64
Potato	16
Potato, cooked with skin	18
Pudding, black	55
Pumpkin	44

Quince	30
Radish	15
Radishes	13
Raspberry	18
Rhubarb	12
Rolls, bread	21
Rye, whole grain	51
Sauerkraut, dripped off	16
Sausage "Bierschincken"	85
Sausage "Fleischwurst"	78
Sausage "Mortadella"	96
Sausage "Munich Weisswurst"	73
Sausage, Vienna	78

Sausages, frying, from veal	91
Sausages, German (Mettwurst)	74
Sesame (gingelly) seed, Oriental, dry	62
Spinach	57
Squash, summer	24
Strawberry	21
Tench	80
Tofu	68
Tomato	11
Nuts, Walnut	25
Wheat, whole grain	51
Yogurt, min. 3.5% fat content	8.1

This Page Has Been Left Blank Intentionally.

Chapter 8

Recipes: 85 Simple & Most Healthy Recipes for Gout

Breakfast Recipes

A MESSAGE FOR READERS

The recipes listed under Breakfast section are extremely healthy and nutritious for Gout. You may or can adjust the quantity of ingredients based on the servings you are preparing.

SIMPLE HOMEMADE YAM FRIES

Yield: 4 servings

Ingredients

2 tbsp. unsalted low-fat butter
1 large shallot (diced)
1 lb. yams (diced)
1/8 tsp. salt
Fresh ground black pepper
¼ tsp. dried thyme leaves
¼ tsp. dried oregano leaves

Directions

1. Start by placing a large skillet in the oven and preheating the oven to 325°F.
2. Once the pan is hot, add yams, shallots and the spread.
3. Now, return the pan into the oven and Let the yams cook for about 10 minutes.
4. Continue to stir and roast the yams in the oven. Stir every 8 to 10 minutes. The yams will begin to soften in about 30 minutes.
5. Now, add the oregano, pepper, salt and thyme. Stir well.
6. Let the yams cook for another 5 to 8 minutes until the yams become slightly crispy on the outside and soft on the inside.

CLASSIC HASH BROWNS

Yield: 2 servings

Ingredients

8 ounces yukon gold potatoes (shredded)
1/8 tsp. salt
Fresh ground black pepper (to taste)
2 tsp. unsalted low-fat butter

Directions

1. Start by shredding the potatoes. Now place the shredded potatoes in a strainer. Remove the excess water from potatoes with the help of a spatula (back of spatula).
2. Next step is to pat dry the potatoes on a thick paper towel. Try to make them as dry as possible.
3. Now, place the shredded potatoes in a bowl and add the pepper and salt. Toss well.
4. Now, take and place a large skillet over medium heat and place butter on it.
5. Once the butter is melted, add the potatoes.
6. Toss the potatoes well and cook for about 5 minutes. Make two piles of potatoes and press then nicely to flatten each potato pile.
7. Cook the potatoes slowly on medium to medium high heat so that they don't burn.
8. Turn and cook on each side for about 5 minutes.
9. Serve immediately.

LOW SODIUM HOME FRIES

Yield: 2 servings

Ingredients

8 ounces red yukon gold potatoes (diced)
Spray oil
1 small onion (diced)
1/8 tsp. salt
Fresh ground black pepper

Directions

1. Take a glass bowl and place the potatoes (diced) in it. Now, microwave the potatoes on high for about 1 minute. Remove from microwave and stir well. Let the potatoes rest for 3 minutes. Repeat this step 2 times.
2. Take and place a large non-stick skillet over medium high heat and spray lightly with cooking oil. Once the skillet is hot, add the onions. Cook the onions until light brown.
3. Once the onions are brown, add the potatoes, pepper and salt. Spray again lightly with cooking oil. Toss the potatoes until they are lightly brown.
4. Serve hot.

HOME FRIES VERSION 2

Yield: 2 servings

Ingredients

8 ounces red or yukon gold potatoes (cut into ¼ inch dice)
Spray oil
1 small onion (diced)
¼ medium red bell pepper (diced)
¼ medium green bell pepper (diced)
1/8 tsp. salt
Fresh ground black pepper (to taste)

Directions

1. Take a glass bowl and place the potatoes (diced) in it. Now, microwave the potatoes on high for about 1 minute. Remove from microwave and stir well. Let the potatoes rest for 3 minutes. Repeat this step 2 times.
2. Take and place a large non-stick skillet over medium high heat and spray lightly with cooking oil. Once the skillet is hot, add the onions. Cook the onions until light brown.
3. Now, add the peppers and cook for 2 minutes. Toss well frequently.
4. Once the onions are brown, add the potatoes, pepper and salt. Spray again lightly with cooking oil. Toss the potatoes until they are lightly brown.
5. Serve hot.

SWEET POTATO HASH BROWNS

Yield: 2 servings

Ingredients

8 ounces sweet potatoes (shredded)
1/8 tsp. salt
1 tsp. dried sage
Fresh ground black pepper (to taste)
2 tsp. unsalted low-fat butter

Directions

1. Start by shredding the potatoes. Now place the shredded potatoes in a strainer. Remove the excess water from potatoes with the help of a spatula (back of spatula).
2. Next step is to pat dry the potatoes on a thick paper towel. Try to make them as dry as possible.
3. Now, place the shredded potatoes in a bowl and add the sage, pepper and salt. Toss well.
4. Now, take and place a large skillet over medium heat and place butter on it.
5. Once the butter is melted, add the potatoes.
6. Toss the potatoes well and cook for about 5 minutes. Make two piles of potatoes and press then nicely to flatten each potato pile.
7. Cook the potatoes slowly on medium to medium high heat so that they don't burn.
8. Turn and cook on each side for about 5 minutes.
9. Serve immediately.

THE BREAKFAST CORNFLAKES

Yield: 1 serving

Ingredients

2 cups cornflakes
1 cup 1% low-fat milk
1 cup berries, fresh or frozen, thawed

Directions

1. Take a small bowl and place cornflakes in it.
2. Top the cornflakes with berries and milk.
3. Serve.

THE BREAKFAST SMOOTHIE

Yield: 2 servings

Ingredients

1 apple
1 pear
½ tsp. freshly grated ginger
2 tbsp. flax seeds (ground right before consumption)
6 large kale leaves (woody stems removed), or 2 handfuls of spinach
Juice of 1 small lemon
1 cup water

Directions

1. Quarter an apple and a pear. Remove the seeds and stems. Place the apple and pear in a blender.
2. Now, add the remaining ingredients to the blender and puree. Add a little more water, if required.

THE BREAKFAST FRUIT SALAD

Yield: 2 servings

Ingredients

2 oranges, peeled and diced
2 apples, diced
1 cup walnuts, chopped (optional)
1 tsp. cinnamon

Directions

1. Take a bowl and add fruits in it.
2. Now, sprinkle the cinnamon and chopped nuts.

THE BREAKFAST MELON SMOOTHIE

Yield: 1-2 servings

Ingredients

3 cups watermelon chunks
1 small ripe banana, chopped
1 cup ice
1 ½ cups of 0% fat vanilla yogurt

Directions

1. Place yogurt, ice, watermelon chunks and chopped banana in the blender. Blend well until the desired smoothness is achieved.
2. Serve.

THE BREAKFAST DATES SHAKE

Yield: 1-2 servings

Ingredients

½ cup corn flakes
3 cups low-fat milk
½ cup pureed dates
4-5 ice cubes

Directions

1. Start by soaking the cornflakes in 1 cup of milk for about 5 minutes.
2. Now, add all the ingredients in a blender and blend until smooth and frothy.
3. Serve immediately.

BANANA AND CINNAMON CORNFLAKES

Yield: 1 serving

Ingredients

1 large ripe banana sliced
1 cup corn flakes
A pinch of cinnamon powder
1 cup warm low-fat milk

Directions

1. Take a bowl and fill it with cornflakes.
2. Now, add warm milk, banana and cinnamon powder. Mix it well.
3. Serve immediately.

CRANBERRY AND ALMONDS CORNFLAKES

Yield: 1 serving

Ingredients

1 cup corn flakes
¼ cup dried cranberries
2 tbsp. chopped almonds
1 ½ cups of cold low-fat milk

Directions

1. Take a bowl and fill it with cornflakes.
2. Now, add the cold milk to cornflakes.
3. Now, top the cornflakes with almonds and cranberries.
4. Serve immediately.

DELICIOUS CINNAMON & APPLE DELIGHT

Yield: 1 serving

Ingredients

6 ounces of non-fat greek yogurt
¼ a teaspoon of vanilla extract
¼ a tablespoon of cinnamon
1 large apple

Directions

1. Take an apple, core it and cut into chunks.
2. Take a small bowl and stir yogurt, stevia (optional, as per taste), cinnamon and vanilla extract.
3. Now, add the apples and toss well to coat.
4. Now, refrigerate for 5-8 minutes before serving.

THE GREEK FRUIT SALAD

Yield: 1 serving

Ingredients

1 tablespoon of honey
2 tablespoons of walnuts
½ a cup of fruits of your choice
4 ounces of no-fat greek yogurt

Directions

1. Take a sundae glass or parfait and layer some of the fruit pieces. Now, top the fruit pieces with yoghurt. Once done, layer more fruits on the top.
2. Now, sprinkle cinnamon and walnuts. Now, drizzle the honey and serve.

THE BERRY BREAKFAST

Yield: 1 serving

Ingredients

1 cup frozen unsweetened raspberries
¾ cup chilled unsweetened almond or rice milk
¼ cup frozen pitted unsweetened cherries or raspberries
1 ½ tbsp. honey
2 tsp. finely grated fresh ginger
1 tsp. ground flaxseed
1-2 tsp. fresh lemon juice

Directions

1. Take a blender and combine all the ingredients in it. Add the lemon juice as per taste.
2. Now, puree everything until smooth.
3. Serve.

Lunch Recipes

A MESSAGE FOR READERS

The recipes listed under Lunch section are extremely healthy and nutritious for Gout. You may or can adjust the quantity of ingredients based on the servings you are preparing.

BROCCOLI AND BROWN RICE PASTA

Yield: 2-3 servings

Ingredients

1 large head broccoli, cut into chunks and florets (peel the stem and cut into chunks)
1 pound brown rice pasta shells
1/3 cup extra-virgin olive oil
2-3 large garlic cloves, minced
Crushed red pepper flakes to taste
Low sodium salt and fresh ground pepper to taste

Directions

1. Start by filling a large pasta pot with low-sodium salted water (about 3/4 full) and bring to a boil. Now, add the pasta shells and bring again to the boil.
2. Now, add the broccoli stem chunks to the pot and let them cook for 1 minute. Next, add the broccoli florets and continue to boil until the pasta is cooked. Now, strain the pasta and return to the pot.
3. In the meanwhile, take and place a large frying pan over medium-high heat. Now, add olive oil, garlic, pepper, red pepper and salt to it. Without letting the garlic burn, continue to heat until sizzling. Once it starts sizzling, pour this mixture on to the pasta and toss well until moist.
4. You may sprinkle a little bit of parmesan cheese on top of the pasta while serving.

BAKED SWEET POTATOS

Yield: 1-2 servings

Ingredients

2 tablespoons olive oil
3 large sweet potatoes
2 pinches dried oregano
2 pinches of low sodium salt
2 pinches of ground black pepper

Directions

1. Start by preheating the oven to 350 degrees F.
2. Take a glass or non-stick baking dish and coat its bottom with olive oil. Use olive oil just enough to coat the bottom.
3. Next step is to wash and peel the sweet potatoes. Once done, cut the sweet potatoes to medium-size pieces.
4. Now, place the sweet potatoes pieces into the baking dish. Turn the pieces nicely to coat them with olive oil.
5. Now, sprinkle salt, pepper and oregano.
6. Now, bake the sweet potatoes in a preheated oven at 350 degrees F for about 60 minutes or until the sweet potatoes are soft.

BAKED SWEET POTATOS WITH GINGER AND HONEY

Yield: 1-2 servings

Ingredients

3 pounds sweet potatoes, peeled and cubed
½ cup honey
3 tablespoons grated fresh ginger
2 tablespoons walnut oil
1 teaspoon ground cardamom
½ teaspoon ground black pepper

Directions

1. Start by preheating the oven to 400 degrees F.
2. Toss together sweet potatoes, walnut oil, honey, cardamom, ginger and pepper in a large bowl. Now transfer everything to a large cast iron frying pan.
3. Now, bake for about 20 minutes in a preheated oven. Make sure to stir in between for even baking.
4. Once you stir, bake for another 20 minutes or so or until the sweet potatoes are soft, tender and nicely caramelized on the outside.

SIMPLE BAKED BROWN RICE

Yield: 2 servings

Ingredients

1 ½ cups brown rice
2 ½ cups water
2 tbsp. of olive oil
1 teaspoon low sodium salt

Directions

1. Start by preheating the oven to 375 degrees F. Next, place the brown rice in an 8 inches square baking dish (glass).
2. Take a saucepan. Add water, salt and olive oil. Bring to a boil. Once the water boils, pour it over the rice in the baking dish and mix well.
3. Now, cover the baking dish tightly with the aluminium foil. Bake the rice on the middle rack of the oven for about an hour.
4. Once done, let it sit for 5 minutes and serve hot.

STIR FRIED KALE

Yield: 1-2 servings

Ingredients

2 tablespoons olive oil
1 onion, chopped
3 cloves garlic, minced
1 cup bread crumbs
3 bunches kale - washed, dried, and shredded

Directions

1. Take a large frying pan and heat oil over medium high heat. Once the oil is hot, add the onions and garlic. Sauté them until soft.
2. Once the onions are soft, add the breadcrumbs. Stir and cook them until brown.
3. Now, add in the kale. Stir and cook until wilted.
4. Serve hot either as is or with brown rice.

BUTTERNUT SQUASH BAKE

Yield: 4-5 servings

Ingredients

6 cups cubed butternut squash
2 tablespoons sesame seeds
2 tablespoons olive oil
1 serrano chili, seeded and chopped
1 teaspoon dried tarragon
1 teaspoon dried basil
1 pinch salt
1 pinch turmeric

Directions

1. Start by preheating the oven to 350°F.
2. Take a baking tray and mix all the ingredients.
3. Once mixed and oven is preheated, place the tray in the oven and bake for about 30 to 40 minutes or until the squash is tender and golden brown on the outside.
4. Serve warm.

QUINOA STUFFED BELL PEPPERS

Yield: 4 servings

Ingredients

4 red bell peppers
3 cups cooked quinoa
¼ cup chopped parsley
¼ cup chopped cilantro
1 shallot, finely chopped
1 ripe tomato, diced
1 pinch turmeric
1 pinch salt
1 pinch black pepper
2 cups water
½ lemon, juiced
½ cup low-fat yogurt to serve

Directions

1. Start with cutting the top off of each bell pepper; remove the core. Make sure to leave the pepper intact.
2. Now, take a bowl and combine the quinoa with cilantro, parsley, shallot, turmeric, salt and black pepper.
3. Mix the mixture well and once done, spoon the mixture into each pepper.
4. Now, place the bell peppers into a deep pan.
5. Now, add water, lemon juice to the pan and cook on a low heat for about 30 minutes.
6. Serve the cooked stuffed peppers with low-fat yogurt.

THE CARROT PILAF

Yield: 4-5 servings

Ingredients

2 tablespoons olive oil
1 shallot, finely chopped
1 garlic clove, chopped
1½ cups pearl barley, rinsed
½ pound baby carrots, sliced
3 cups low-sodium vegetable stock
2 tablespoons chopped parsley
1 pinch salt
1 pinch black pepper

Directions

1. Take a heavy saucepan and heat the oil. Once the oil is hot, add the shallot and garlic.
2. Sauté the shallot and garlic for about 2 minutes and then add the barley. Stir and sauté for another 2 minutes.
3. Now, add carrots and the vegetable stock. Cook the pilaf for about 30 minutes on a low heat.
4. Now, add salt, black pepper and parsley. Stir well.
5. Serve warm.

GINGER CARROT SOUP

Yield: 2-4 servings

Ingredients

1 tablespoon olive oil
1 shallot, chopped
1 garlic clove, chopped
1½ pounds baby carrots
2 cups low-sodium vegetable stock
2 cups water
1 tablespoon grated ginger
½ teaspoon dried thyme
1 pinch turmeric
1 pinch black pepper

Directions

1. Take a soup pot and heat oil in it. Once the oil is hot, stir in the shallot and garlic. Sauté the shallot and garlic for about 2 minutes and then add the carrots.
2. Let cook for about 5 more minutes and then pour the vegetable stock, water and also add thyme, ginger, black pepper and turmeric.
3. Let cook the soup for about 30 minutes on low heat.
4. Once done, purée the ginger carrot soup with the help of an immersion blender.
5. Serve immediately.

SIMPLE ONION SOUP

Yield: 4-6 servings

Ingredients

3 large onions, sliced
4 shallots, sliced
4 tablespoons olive oil
1 tablespoon dried rosemary
1 teaspoon dried thyme
2 cups water
4 cups low-sodium stock
1 pinch black pepper
4-6 slices white bread
4 thin slices low-fat cheese

Directions

1. Take a soup pot and heat oil in it. Once the oil is hot, stir in the shallot and garlic. Sauté the shallot and garlic for about 20 minutes until the onions are caramelized.
2. Now, add thyme, rosemary, black pepper and then the water and vegetable stock.
3. Let the soup cook for about 30 minutes on a medium heat.
4. Now, pour the onion soup into the individual bowls and top the bowls with a bread slice and cheese.
5. Now, place these bowls under a broiler and cook for about 5 to10 minutes until the cheese melts.
6. Serve the onion soup warm.

BROWN RICE PASTA WITH CHICKEN

Note: As poultry is moderately high in purine, the serving size should not exceed **3 ounces or 85 grams per day**. You can enjoy chicken as a side dish or main dish with a healthy salad.

Yield: 2 servings

Ingredients

Brown rice pasta shells as per requirement
1 teaspoon olive oil
2 cloves garlic, minced
1 boneless, skinless chicken breast, cut into bite-size pieces
Crushed red pepper flakes to taste
1/3 cup oil-packed sun-dried tomatoes, drained and cut into strips
Low sodium pasta sauce (use any as per taste but in very little quantity)

Directions

1. Take a large pot and fill it with low-sodium salted water and bring to a boil. Now, add the pasta and cook for about 8-10 minutes or until pasta is cooked. Now, drain the water and set aside.
2. Take a large skillet and heat oil over medium heat. Add and sauté the garlic until it is tender. Once the garlic is tender, add and stir in the chicken. Add red pepper flakes and cook the chicken golden in colour or cooked completely.
3. Take a large bowl and combine, chicken, pasta, pasta sauce and sun-dried tomatoes. Toss well to coat nicely.

QUINOA WITH BLACK BEANS

Yield: 4-6 servings

Ingredients

1 teaspoon vegetable oil
1 onion, chopped
3 cloves garlic, chopped
¾ cup quinoa
1 ½ cups vegetable broth
1 teaspoon ground cumin
¼ teaspoon cayenne pepper
Low sodium salt and ground black pepper to taste
1 cup frozen corn kernels
2 (15 ounce) cans black beans, rinsed and drained
½ cup chopped fresh cilantro

Directions

1. Take a saucepan and heat oil over medium heat. Add the onion and garlic. Stir and cook until lightly browned.
2. Now, add the quinoa into the onion mixture. Add the vegetable broth. Add cayenne pepper, salt, cumin and pepper. Now, bring this mixture to a boil. Reduce the heat, cover and simmer until the quinoa is tender and vegetable broth is absorbed well, This may take about 20 minutes.
3. Add the frozen corn to the quinoa, and continue to cook for about 5 minutes (on low heat).
4. Finally, add and stir well the cilantro and black beans.

SPRING ONIONS & SQUASH

Yield: 3 servings

Ingredients

2 cups yellow straight neck or crook neck squash, washed and sliced
2 tablespoons low-fat or 0% fat margarine
1 cup green onion, chopped
1 teaspoon black pepper

Directions

1. Start by boiling the squash slices for about 15 minutes or until tender. Drain.
2. Take a frying pan and melt the butter. Sauté the spring onions for about one minute.
3. Now, stir in the squash and black pepper.
4. Cover the pan and allow it to simmer on low heat for about 5 minutes.
5. Serve hot.

OVEN BAKED YELLOW SQUASH

Yield: 6 servings

Ingredients

2 tablespoons margarine or butter, melted
¾ teaspoon thyme
⅛ teaspoon black pepper
2 cans yellow squash, sliced
1 medium onion, chopped
1 small stalk celery, chopped
1 large bell pepper, chopped
1 tablespoon lemon juice

Directions

1. Start by preheating the oven to 350°F.
2. Next step is to sauté all the ingredients except the lemon juice in margarine. Cook until the onions become translucent.
3. Now, add the lemon juice.
4. Now, place the sautéed mixture in a casserole dish.
5. Finally, bake it for about 30 minutes.
6. Serve hot.

WHITE RICE O'BRIEN

Yield: 4 servings

Ingredients

1½ cup water
1 cup uncooked white rice
½ cup spring onions, finely chopped
¼ cup carrots, shredded
¼ tsp. paprika
½ tsp. black pepper, ground
½ tsp. dry thyme
1 tbsp. fresh lemon juice
1 tbsp. low-fat margarine

Directions

1. Take a large saucepan and boil water in it. In the boiling water, combine all ingredients.
2. Cover the pan and let it simmer for about 15 minutes without stirring.
3. Now, remove from the pan and fluff the rice lightly with the help of a fork.

Dinner Recipes

A MESSAGE FOR READERS

The recipes listed under Dinner section are extremely healthy and nutritious for Gout. You may or can adjust the quantity of ingredients based on the servings you are preparing.

ZUCCHINI LASAGNA STEW

Yield: 4-5 servings

Ingredients

4 zucchinis, cubed
1 onion, chopped
1 garlic clove, chopped
1 tablespoon olive oil
1 green bell pepper, cored and diced
1 red bell pepper, cored and diced
2 cups tomato sauce
¼ cup water
½ teaspoon cumin powder
1 pinch salt
1 pinch black pepper
2 tablespoons chopped cilantro

Directions

1. Take a heavy saucepan and heat oil. Add the onion and garlic. Sauté the onion and garlic for about 2 minutes.
2. Now, stir in the zucchinis and bell peppers, Continue to sauté for about 5 minutes, stirring often.
3. Now, add the remaining ingredients, except cilantro, and cook for 30 minutes on low heat.
4. Once done, remove from heat and add chopped cilantro. Stir well.
5. Serve warm.

QUINOA RATATOUILLE

Yield: 4-5 servings

Ingredients

1 large eggplant, peeled and cubed
1 large zucchini, cubed
2 red bell peppers, cored and cubed
2 ripe tomatoes, cubed
2 garlic cloves, chopped
1 red onion, chopped
1 tablespoon olive oil
3 cups vegetable stock
½ cup couscous
1 teaspoon dried thyme
1 teaspoon dried rosemary
2 tablespoons chopped cilantro
2 tablespoons chopped parsley
1 pinch salt
1 pinch black pepper
1 pinch cumin powder
1 pinch turmeric
½ teaspoon celery seeds

Directions

1. Start by combining eggplant, bell peppers, tomatoes, zucchini, onion and garlic in a large heavy pot.
2. Now, add oil and vegetable stock. Cook for 20 minutes on a medium heat.
3. Now, add the couscous, stir well and cook for about 20 more minutes.
4. Now, add the celery seeds, salt, black pepper, rosemary,

thyme, turmeric, cumin and then remove from heat, stir in the remaining herbs (chopped).
5. Serve warm.

THE VEGETABLE STEW

Yield: 6-8 servings

Ingredients

2 tablespoons coconut oil
2 eggplants, peeled and cubed
1 large zucchini, cubed
1 pumpkin, cubed
2 tomatoes, diced
1 red onion, chopped
1 can chickpeas, drained
¼ cup golden raisins
1 cup low-sodium vegetable stock
1 cup water
1 bay leaf
½ teaspoon cumin seeds
1 pinch salt
1 pinch black pepper
¼ cup chopped cilantro

Directions

1. Take a heavy pot and heat oil. Once the oil is hot, add onion. Stir and sauté for about 2 minutes. Now, add the remaining vegetables.
2. Let it cook for about 10 minutes and then add the raisins. Stir well.
3. Now, add the vegetable stock and water. Next, stir in the cumin seeds, bay leaf, salt, and black pepper.
4. Reduce the heat and let cook for about 40 minutes.
5. Once done, remove the stew from heat and add the cilantro. Stir well.

6.   Serve warm.

DELICIOUS STUFFED EGGPLANTS

Yield: 3-4 servings

Ingredients

4 large eggplants cut in half lengthwise
2 tablespoons olive oil
1 shallot, chopped
2 ripe tomatoes
2 teaspoons Italian seasoning
4 basil leaves, chopped
½ cup low-fat mozzarella
1 pinch salt
1 pinch black pepper

Directions

1. Start by scooping out the flesh of eggplants. Once done, chop the eggplants finely. Please make sure that the skins of eggplants remain intact.
2. Take a skillet and heat the oil. Once the oil is hot, add the shallot. Stir and sauté the shallot for about 2 minutes. Now, add tomatoes, eggplant flesh, basil and seasoning.
3. Now, season with salt and black pepper. Sauté for another10 minutes.
4. Now, spoon the eggplant flesh mixture into the eggplant skins. Top with mozzarella cheese.
5. Now, place the eggplant on a baking tray and bake them in a preheated oven at 350°F for about 40 minutes.
6. Serve warm.

SAUTÉED CABBAGE

Yield: 1-2 servings

Ingredients

3 tablespoons olive oil
½ head red cabbage, chopped
½ onion, chopped
1 small red bell pepper, chopped
1 small yellow bell pepper, chopped
Low sodium salt and ground black pepper to taste

Directions

1. Take a large skillet and heat olive oil over high heat.
2. Now, stir and cook the cabbage, red bell pepper, onion and yellow bell pepper in the oil. Stir every 30 seconds until tender for about 5 to 7 minutes in total.
3. Season with salt and black pepper.

BASIC SAUTÉED KALE

Yield: 1-2 servings

Ingredients

1 tablespoon extra-virgin olive oil
1 pound kale, ribs removed, coarsely chopped
½ cup water
1 teaspoon extra-virgin olive oil
2 cloves garlic, minced
¼ teaspoon crushed red pepper
2 teaspoons sherry vinegar or red-wine vinegar
¼ teaspoon low sodium salt

Directions

1. Start by heating 1 tablespoon of oil in a Dutch oven on medium heat.
2. Now, add the kale. Cook kale by tossing it with the help of two large spoons until it gets the bright green colour. This may take about 1 minute.
3. Add water. Now, reduce the heat to medium low. Now, cover and cook (stirring occasionally) for about 12 – 15 minutes or until the kale is tender.
4. Now, push the kale to one side of the Dutch oven. Add 1 teaspoon of oil to the empty side of oven.
5. Add and cook the garlic and crushed red pepper on this side for about 1 minute.
6. Now, remove it from the heat. Add and stir in the vinegar to taste and salt.

SAUTÉED KALE WITH APPLES

Yield: 1-2 servings

Ingredients

1 tablespoon olive oil
1 white onion, sliced
2 red delicious apples, cored and cut into bite-size pieces
2 teaspoons apple cider vinegar
1/8 teaspoon low sodium salt
1/8 teaspoon ground black pepper
4 cups chopped kale leaves

Directions

1. Take a large skillet and heat olive oil over medium heat.
2. Add the onion. Sauté the onion until tender or about 4 minutes.
3. Now, add the apples, salt, pepper and vinegar. Now, cover and cook until apples are tender. This may take about 3 minutes.
4. Finally, add the kale. Cover and cook until the kale is tender. This may take about 4 to 5 minutes.
5. Serve hot.

ROASTED BEETS AND SAUTÉED BEET GREENS

Yield: 1-2 servings

Ingredients

1 bunch beets with greens
¼ cup olive oil, divided
2 cloves garlic, minced
2 tablespoons chopped onion (optional)
Low sodium salt and pepper to taste
1 tablespoon red wine vinegar (optional)

Directions

1. Start by preheating the oven to 350 degrees F.
2. Next step is to wash the beets thoroughly. Make sure to leave the skins of beets on but remove the greens. Remove any large stems from the greens and set aside.
3. Now, take a small roasting pan or baking dish and toss it with 2 tablespoons of olive oil.
4. Now, cover and bake the beets for about 45 - 60 minutes or until a toothpick or knife can easily slide inside the largest beet.
5. When the beets are almost roasted, take another skillet and heat the remaining 2 tablespoons of olive oil over medium-low heat.
6. Add the onion and garlic and sauté for a about a minute. Break the greens into 2 to 3 inch pieces, and add them to the hot skillet.
7. Now, stir and cook the greens until wilted and tender.

8. Season with salt and pepper.
9. Serve the beet greens as is. For roasted beets, slice them and serve with butter (season with salt and pepper)

SPICY BUTTERNUT SQUASH SOUP

Yield: 4-5 servings

Ingredients

2 tablespoons olive oil
1 small shallot, chopped
2 garlic cloves, chopped
4 cups cubed butternut squash
½ red chili, chopped
4 cups low-sodium vegetable stock
1 pinch turmeric
1 pinch salt
1 pinch black pepper
½ cup low-fat sour cream

Directions

1. Take a soup pot and heat oil in it. Once the oil is hot, add the shallot and garlic. Cook the shallot and garlic together for about 2 minutes. Now, add the chilli and squash.
2. Now, pour in the vegetable stock. Also, add a pinch of salt, turmeric and black pepper to taste.
3. Let the soup cook for about 30 minutes on a low heat.
4. Once the soup is cooked, purée the soup with the help of an immersion blender. Once done, add the sour cream, stir well and bring the soup to a boil.
5. Remove the soup from the heat and serve warm.

HERBS & VEGGIES RICE CASSEROLE

Yield: 8 servings

Ingredients

1 cup white rice, uncooked
2 cups homemade vegetable stock, unsalted
½ cup zucchini, fresh and finely chopped
½ cup carrots, fresh and finely chopped
½ tsp. parsley flakes
1 tbsp. olive oil
½ cup spring onions, finely chopped
1 tbsp. chives, dry

Directions

1. Start by preheating the oven to 350ºF.
2. Next step is to combine all the ingredients and place in casserole dish.
3. Finally, bake in a covered casserole for about 45 to 50 minutes or until the liquid is absorbed.

OVEN BAKED BUTTERNUT SQUASH

Yield: 4 servings

Ingredients

1 medium butternut squash
1-2 per cube, butter sprays
As per taste, salt
As per taste, ground pepper

Directions

1. Start by chopping the stalk off and flower end. Now, chop it in cubes. Take a spoon and also remove the seeds.
2. Place the squash cubes in a 13x9 baking dish and pour in 1/4 inch of water.
3. Finally, cover and bake at 350ºF for about 45 minutes or until the squash is tender.

SIMPLE LEMON HERB CHICKEN

Note: As poultry is moderately high in purine, the serving size should not exceed **3 ounces or 85 grams per day**. You can enjoy chicken as a side dish or main dish with a healthy salad.

Yield: 2 servings, 3 ounces/serving

Ingredients

2 skinless, boneless chicken breast halves
1 lemon
Low sodium salt and pepper to taste
1 tablespoon olive oil
1 pinch dried oregano
2 sprigs fresh parsley, for garnish

Directions

1. Take a bowl big enough to hold the chicken. Squeeze the juice of half lemon on the chicken. Also, season it with salt. Let the chicken rest for about 15 to 20 minutes.
2. Take a small skillet and heat oil in it over medium–low heat.
3. Once the oil is hot, put chicken in the skillet. While sautéing the chicken, add the juice of other half lemon, oregano and pepper to taste. Sauté for another 5-10 minutes on each side, or until the juices run clear.
4. Garnish the chicken with parsley and serve hot.

GRILLED LEMON CHICKEN

Note: As poultry is moderately high in purine, the serving size should not exceed **3 ounces or 85 grams per day**. You can enjoy chicken as a side dish or main dish with a healthy salad.

Yield: 4 servings, 3 ounces/serving

Ingredients

1/3 cup lemon juice
¼ cup olive oil
1 tablespoon Dijon mustard
2 large cloves garlic, finely chopped
2 tablespoons finely chopped red bell pepper
½ teaspoon low sodium salt
¼ teaspoon ground black pepper
4 skinless, boneless chicken breast halves

Directions

1. Take a large bowl and combine, olive oil, lemon juice Dijon mustard, red bell pepper, garlic, salt and pepper. Reserve and set aside about ¼ cup of this mixture.
2. Take a bowl big enough to hold the chicken. Now, coat the chicken with the mixture well. Refrigerate the marinated chicken for a minimum of 20 to 30 minutes.
3. Next step is to pre-heat the grill on high heat.
4. Now, oil the grill grate lightly and place the marinated chicken on the grill. Let the chicken cook for 6 to 8 minutes on each side or until the juices run clear. Keep basting the chicken occasionally with the reserved marinade.

SPRING ONIONS AND HERBS CHICKEN CURRY

Note: As poultry is moderately high in purine, the serving size should not exceed **3 ounces or 85 grams per day**. You can enjoy chicken as a side dish or main dish with a healthy salad.

Yield: 6 servings, 3 ounces/serving

Ingredients

1 whole chicken, skin removed and cut into small pieces
¼ cup lemon juice
2 tsps. curry powder
½ cup spring onions, finely chopped
½ tsp. black pepper
½ tsp. thyme, dry
2 tbsp. olive oil
1 cup water

Directions

1. Start by cleaning the whole chicken and cut into small pieces.
2. Once you cut the chicken into small pieces, give the chicken pieces a bath of lemon juice.
3. Next, take a medium sized bowl and combine spring onions, curry powder, black pepper, thyme together. Once combined, rub the mixture onto the chicken pieces.
4. Next step is to let the chicken marinate in the refrigerator overnight or at least for 1 to 2 hours.
5. Take a sauce pan and heat the vegetable oil. Sauté the

marinated chicken until it turns brown.

6. Once the chicken turns brown, pour one cup of water into the pan and let the chicken simmer until it gets tender.

7. Once the chicken becomes tender, remove it from the heat and serve with hot rice.

OLD STYLE RICE AND CHICKEN

Note: As poultry is moderately high in purine, the serving size should not exceed **3 ounces or 85 grams per day**. You can enjoy chicken as a side dish or main dish with a healthy salad.

Yield: 6 servings, ¾ cup, 3 ounces chicken/serving

Ingredients

1 pound chicken, cut into pieces
½ tsp. black pepper, ground
1 tbsp. poultry seasoning
½ cup spring onions, chopped
½ tsp. onion powder
2-3 crushed bay leaves (optional)
4 cups water
1 cup white rice, uncooked
1 tbsp. olive oil

Directions

1. Take a Dutch oven covered with water and put the chicken pieces, spring onions, onion powder, black pepper, poultry seasoning and bay leaves.
2. Cook the chicken until tender.
3. Once the chicken is cooked, remove the chicken meat and skin from the bone. Keep the chicken meat but discard the skin. Also reserve 2 cups of chicken broth.
4. Take a large pot and put rice, vegetable oil, chicken meat and 2 cups of chicken broth in it. Now, bring it to a boil over medium-high heat.

5.   Once it comes to a boil, reduce the heat to low and simmer for about 20 to 25 minutes.
6.   Serve hot.

Salads Recipes

A MESSAGE FOR READERS

The recipes listed under Salads section are extremely healthy and nutritious for Gout. You may or can adjust the quantity of ingredients based on the servings you are preparing.

THE WALDORF SALAD

Yield: 2-4 servings

Ingredients

2 green apples, peeled and diced
1 cup seedless red grapes
2 celery stalks, sliced
6 lettuce leaves, shredded
1 tablespoon lemon juice
2 tablespoons low-fat mayonnaise
2 tablespoons plain yogurt
1 pinch black pepper
10 walnuts

Directions

1. Take a salad bowl and combine apples, celery, lettuce and grapes together.
2. Now, add mayonnaise, yogurt, walnuts, black pepper and lemon juice. Mix well gently.
3. Serve fresh.

THE COUSCOUS SALAD

Yield: 4-6 servings

Ingredients

1 cup couscous, rinsed
3 cups hot vegetable stock
1 cucumber, sliced
2 ripe tomatoes, cubed
1 shallot, sliced
½ cup chopped parsley
½ cup chopped cilantro
4 mint leaves, chopped
1 pinch salt
1 pinch black pepper
½ lemon, juiced

Directions

1. Take a bowl and combine couscous and hot vegetable stock. Cover the lid and let the couscous absorb the stock for about 20 minutes. Once done, use a fork to fluff it up.
2. Now, stir in the tomatoes, cucumber, parsley, cilantro, shallot and mint.
3. Now, add salt, pepper and lemon juice. Mix well gently.
4. Serve fresh.

THE ZUCCHINI SALAD

Yield: 2-4 servings

Ingredients

2 zucchinis, finely sliced
1 red chili, seeded and sliced
½ teaspoon mustard powder
½ lemon, juiced
1 cup coarsely chopped parsley
¼ cup chopped cilantro
6 mint leaves, chopped
1 pinch salt
1 pinch black pepper

Directions

1. Take a bowl and combine zucchinis, cilantro, parsley, mint and chilli.
2. Now, add salt, black pepper, mustard powder and lemon juice. Stir well gently.
3. Serve fresh.

THE TOMATO AND BREAD SALAD

Yield: 4-6 servings

Ingredients

2 pounds heirloom tomatoes, cubed
4 slices whole wheat bread, cubed
2 tablespoons chopped basil
1 cucumber, sliced
½ cup pitted black olives
½ cup cubed low-fat mozzarella
1 tablespoon balsamic vinegar
1 pinch salt
1 pinch black pepper
½ teaspoon dried oregano

Directions

1. Take a bowl and combine cucumber, tomatoes, black olives, vinegar, basil, mozzarella, oregano, salt and pepper. Mix well gently.
2. Now, stir in the bread.
3. Serve fresh.

ARUGULA AND PEAR SALAD

Yield: 4-6 servings

Ingredients

4 cups arugula leaves
2 ripe pears, finely sliced
½ lemon, juiced
1 tablespoon olive oil
1 tablespoon Dijon mustard
1 pinch black pepper

Directions

1. Start by placing the arugula on a platter and then top it with the pear slices.
2. Take a small sized jar and combine lemon juice, mustard, olive oil and black pepper. Now, cover the lid of the jar and shake the ingredients well.
3. Pour this dressing over the salad. Mix well gently.
4. Serve fresh.

THE AVOCADO KALE SALAD

Yield: 2 servings

Ingredients

1 medium bunch kale (any type), stemmed and shredded
1 avocado, pitted and flesh removed
1 lemon, juiced

Directions

1.   Take a bowl and combine kale, lemon juice and avocado. Use your hands or any other tool to cream the avocado until mixed well.
2.   Season with salt and pepper to taste. Toss well.
3.   Serve fresh.

CANTALOUPE AND KALE SALAD

Yield: 2 servings

Ingredients

½ large cantaloupe, diced
1 bunch kale, chopped
2 tablespoons olive oil
1 tablespoon white vinegar
½ teaspoon salt

Directions

1. Take a large bowl and combine kale, olive oil, cantaloupe, vinegar and salt together.
2. Toss well gently.
3. Serve fresh.

KALE WALDORF SALAD

Yield: 5 servings

Ingredients

4 cups chopped kale
1 cucumber, chopped
½ cup walnuts, halved

Ingredients for the dressing

2 tbsp. Dijon mustard
1 tbsp. red wine vinegar
2 tbsp. water

Directions

1. Tear the kale into small sized pieced and place into a bowl. Now, massage the kale with your hands until the kale get a bright green colour. This may take about 3 minutes. Once done, add in the chopped cucumber.
2. Take another bowl and combine all the dressing ingredients. Mix well. Now, pour the dressing over cucumber and kale. Toss well.
3. Add walnuts. Toss well.
4. Serve fresh.

PASTA CABBAGE SALAD

Yield: 4-6 servings

Ingredients

3 cups gemelli pasta
3 cups shredded red cabbage
2 medium carrots, shredded
1 ½ cups creamy roasted garlic salad dressing

Directions

1. Take a large pan and boil water in it. Now, cook the rotini as per the directions given on the package. Drain.
2. In the meanwhile, take a large bowl and combine all the remaining ingredients together. Once done, add in the cooked and drained rotini pasta. Stir gently.
3. Chill for about 2 to 3 hours before serving the salad.

THE AVOCADO POTATO SALAD

Yield: 6 servings

Ingredients

1 ½ lbs. red potatoes (cut into ½ inch dice)
2 cups water
1 small avocado
2 ribs celery (diced)
1 small shallot (minced)
¼ tsp. salt
½ tsp. cumin
Fresh ground black pepper (to taste)

Directions

1. Take a large sauce pan and place a steamer basket on it. Add water and set the heat on high.
2. Once the water boils, place in the red potatoes to the steamer basket and steam until tender (about 15-18 minutes).
3. Once done, remove the basket and run through the cold water to stop the cooking process or until the potatoes are at room temperature.
4. Take a bowl and combine potatoes, celery, avocado, shallot, cumin, salt and pepper. Fold gently.
5. Chill well and serve.

BEETS AND SHALLOTS SALAD

Yield: 4 servings

Ingredients

1 lb. yellow beets
8 ounces shallots (peeled)
1 tsp. olive oil
½ tsp. lemon zest
2 tsp. coarse ground mustard
¼ tsp. salt
Fresh ground black pepper (to taste)
1 tsp. fresh thyme leaves
2 tbsp. pine nuts (pignoles)

Directions

1. Start by preheating the oven to 325°F.
2. Wash and scrub the beets well and wrap them each in a foil. Once done, place the wrapped beets into the oven.
3. Take a medium size sauce pan, add oil and shallots. Now, cover the pan and place in the oven.
4. Let the shallots and beets roast for about 50 minutes. Once roasted, remove from the oven and let cool.
5. Once cool, peel and cut the beets into 1/3 inch dice size and place them in a medium size bowl.
6. Now, combine shallots and the liquid from the roast pan with the beets.
7. Finally, add the mustard, thyme, pine nuts, lemon zest, salt and pepper. Toss well.
8. Chill and serve.

THE GREEK QUINOA SALAD

Yield: 2 servings

Ingredients

2 cups water
½ cup quinoa
1 small shallot (minced)
1 tbsp. olive oil
2 medium ribs celery (diced)
½ medium green bell pepper (diced)
4 ounces grape tomatoes (halved)
1 tbsp. capers
1 tbsp. white wine vinegar
2 ounces feta cheese (finely diced or crumbled)
1/8 tsp. salt
Fresh ground black pepper (to taste)
2 tbsp. Italian parsley (chopped)

Directions

1. Start by boiling the water in a small sauce pan.
2. Once the water boils, add the quinoa. Let it cook on high simmer heat with partially covered pan. Let it cook until the water is almost evaporated. Make sure to stir occasionally. Turn off the heat and cover the sauce pan once the quinoa is done.
3. After about 5 to 6 minutes, take a bowl and empty the quinoa in it.
4. Now, add the shallot (minced) to the bowl and fold gently. Once done, refrigerate it.
5. Once the quinoa is cool, add celery, tomatoes, pepper, capers, olives, feta cheese, vinegar, parsley, olive oil, salt and pepper.

Fold well.
6.   Chill and serve.

THE GREEN QUINOA SALAD

Yield: 4 servings

Ingredients

2 cups water
1 cup quinoa
2 green onions
½ medium green bell pepper (finely diced)
½ cup parsley (minced)
2 tbsp. olive oil
1 tbsp. white wine vinegar
¼ tsp. salt
Fresh ground black pepper (to taste)

Directions

1. Start by boiling the water in a small sauce pan. Once the water boils, add the quinoa.
2. Once the water boils, add the quinoa. Let it cook on high simmer heat with partially covered pan. Let it cook until the water is almost evaporated. Make sure to stir occasionally. Turn off the heat and cover the sauce pan once the quinoa is done. Once done, refrigerate it.
3. While the quinoa is being cooking, remove the green part of the onions.
4. Now, cut or slice the white portion of the onions in half lengthwise and then crosswise. Repeat this process with the green tops too.
5. Once the quinoa is cool, combine it in a bowl with green pepper, green onions, olive oil, vinegar, parsley, salt and pepper. Toss well.
6. Serve chill.

THE PURPLE POTATOES SALAD

Yield: 4 servings

Ingredients

1 lb. purple potatoes
Spray grapeseed oil
¼ tsp. salt
Fresh ground black pepper
2 tbsp. olive oil
4 tsp. balsamic vinegar
2 tbsp. fresh dill
2 small ribs celery with leaves

Directions

1. Take a large skillet and place it in the oven. Now, preheat the oven to 325°F.
2. Once the oven is hot, spray the pan lightly with cooking oil. Now, place the potatoes on the pan and back into the oven. Roast the potatoes for 20 to 25 minutes or until the potatoes are tender.
3. Once done, remove the pan and let it cool.
4. Once cool, slice the potatoes into about ½ inch thick slices.
5. Now, take a bowl and combine potatoes with olive oil, balsamic vinegar, diced celery, dill, salt and pepper. Fold well gently.
6. Chill and serve.

THE ROASTED EGGPLANTS SALAD

Yield: 8 servings

Ingredients

Spray olive oil
2 medium eggplants (cut into ½ inch cubes)
2 medium yellow onions (cut into 1/8 wedges)
1 pint grape tomatoes
¼ cup slivered almonds
½ tsp. salt
Fresh ground black pepper
2 tbsp. extra virgin olive oil
3 tbsp. balsamic vinegar
¼ cup fresh basil (chiffonade)
1 tbsp. fresh oregano
1 bulb roasted garlic (chopped)

Directions

1. Take a large skillet and place it in the oven. Now, preheat the oven to 325°F.
2. Once the oven is hot, spray the pan lightly with cooking oil. Now, place the eggplant, tomatoes, almonds and onions on the pan and back into the oven. Roast for about 30 to 40 minutes.
3. Stir the veggies in every 10 minutes. If you find them sticking to the pan, spray the oil once or twice, as needed.
4. Once done, remove the pan from the oven and let the vegetables cool.
5. Once cool, take a bowl and combine the veggies with oregano, basil, roasted garlic, olive oil, vinegar, salt and pepper.
6. Chill and serve.

Dips Recipes

A MESSAGE FOR READERS

The recipes listed under Dips section are extremely healthy and nutritious for Gout. You may or can adjust the quantity of ingredients based on the servings you are preparing.

SIMPLE CHICKPEA DIP

Yield: 2-4 servings

Ingredients

1 can chickpeas, drained
2 garlic cloves
2 tablespoons tahini paste
½ cup low-fat yogurt
½ teaspoon dried oregano
1 pinch chili flakes
1 pinch salt
1 pinch cumin powder

Directions

1. Combine all of the ingredients in a blender.
2. Blend until smooth.
3. Transfer to a bowl with the help of a spoon.
4. Serve.

SIMPLE YOGURT DIP

Yield: 2-4 servings

Ingredients

1 cup plain yogurt
2 tablespoons chopped shallots
1 tablespoon melted coconut oil
2 tablespoons chopped dill
2 tablespoons chopped chives
Salt and pepper to taste
1 pinch cumin powder

Directions

1. Take a small bowl and combine all the ingredients. Mix well.
2. Now, season with salt and pepper.
3. Serve.

ROASTED GARLIC DIP

Yield: 4-5 servings

Ingredients

4 heads garlic
1 cup low-fat yogurt
½ cup light sour cream
2 tablespoons chopped chives
1 pinch black pepper

Directions

1. Start by cutting the heads of garlic in half lengthwise. Once done, wrap each garlic half in the aluminium foil.
2. Now roast in a preheated oven at 375°F for about 40 minutes.
3. Once done, remove the garlic from the oven. Once warm enough to handle, scoop the soft garlic out.
4. Take a bowl, place garlic in it and mash well. Now, stir in the sour cream, yogurt, chives and black pepper.
5. Mix well and serve.

THE AROMATIC DIP

Yield: 2-4 servings

Ingredients

1 ripe avocado, peeled
2 garlic cloves
½ cup buttermilk
2 tablespoons lemon juice
1 pinch salt
2 green onions, finely chopped
¼ cup chopped parsley
¼ cup chopped cilantro
1 tablespoon chopped tarragon

Directions

1. Combine buttermilk, avocado, lemon juice, garlic and salt in a blender.
2. Blend until smooth
3. Add in the onions and herbs. Stir well.
4. Transfer to a bowl with the help of a spoon.
5. Serve.

THE DELIGHT DIP

Yield: 4-5 servings

Ingredients

1 cup cashews, soaked over night
1 cup coconut flesh
½ cup coconut water
¼ cup olive oil
1 teaspoon turmeric powder
2 teaspoons grated ginger
2 tablespoons maple syrup
1 tablespoon chopped cilantro
Salt, pepper
Carrot, bell pepper, sweet potato and celery sticks

Directions

1. In a food processor, combine coconut flesh, soaked cashews, coconut water, turmeric, maple syrup, olive oil and ginger. Pulse until smooth and creamy.
2. Add in salt, pepper and chopped cilantro. Stir well.
3. Transfer to a bowl with the help of a spoon.
4. Sprinkle with sesame seeds.
5. Serve.

Snacks Recipes

A MESSAGE FOR READERS

The recipes listed under Snacks section are extremely healthy and nutritious for Gout. You may or can adjust the quantity of ingredients based on the servings you are preparing.

SIMPLE BAKED POTATO WEDGES

Yield: 4-6 servings

Ingredients

4 large potatoes
¼ cup cooking oil
1 tablespoon parmesan cheese
1 teaspoon salt
1 tablespoon paprika
½ teaspoon pepper
½ teaspoon garlic powder

Directions

1. Start by washing the potatoes and cut them into wedges.
2. Next step is to place the potatoes (skin down) in the baking dish.
3. Take a small bowl and mix the next six ingredients together. Once mixed, brush the mix onto the potatoes.
4. Bake in the oven at 350 degrees F for about 1 hour.

THE ZUCCHINI ROLLS

Yield: 4 servings

Ingredients

1 large zucchini, finely sliced lengthwise
2 celery stalks, cut into sticks
½ lemon, juiced
1 tablespoon olive oil
1 pinch salt
1 pinch black pepper

Directions

1.   Take a bowl and combine zucchini with salt and black pepper. Drizzle with oil and lemon juice.
2.   Next step is to heat the grill pan over medium heat. Once hot, place the slices of zucchini on to the grill.
3.   Let them cook on both the sides for about 3 to 4 minutes or until browned and tender.
4.   Now, remove the slices of zucchini from the pan and lay them on a chopping board.
5.   Place a few celery sticks at one end of a zucchini slice and roll it tightly. Use a toothpick to secure it. Repeat the same process for the remaining slices.
6.   Serve on a platter fresh.

THE POTATO GRATIN

Yield: 6 servings

Ingredients

6 large white potatoes, peeled
4-6 cloves garlic, sliced
6 sage leaves
Leaves from one sprig of thyme
4 tablespoons olive oil
Salt, freshly ground black pepper

Directions

1. Start by preheating the oven to 340 degrees F.
2. Cut the potatoes to very thin slices but not all the way. Cut through the potato but make sure that the base remains intact. Now, place the potatoes in an oven pan lined with the parchment paper.
3. Next step is to insert the slices of garlic in the slits. Also add a sage leaf to each and every potato.
4. Next, sprinkle some thyme leaves and rub the potatoes with some olive oil. At the end, season the potatoes with some salt and black pepper. Now, cover the oven pan with an aluminium foil.
5. Bake in the preheated oven for about one hour or until the potatoes are completely cooked or tender.

CHICKPEA AND ROASTED EGGPLANT HUMMUS

Yield: 4-6 servings

Ingredients

1 large eggplant, halved
1 can chickpeas, rinsed and drained
3 garlic cloves
2 tablespoons tahini paste
1 pinch black pepper
1 shallot, finely chopped

Directions

1. Start by preheating your oven to 400°F. Once the oven is preheated, take a baking tray and place the eggplant halves on it. Now, bake for about 20 to 25 minutes or until the eggplant halves are soft and browned.
2. Once done, remove eggplants from the oven and scoop the eggplant flesh out.
3. Place the eggplant flesh in a blender. Now, add garlic, chickpeas, tahini paste and black pepper. Pulse until smooth.
4. Transfer the hummus to a bowl and add the chopped shallot. Stir well.
5. Serve fresh.

RICH CHICKPEA HUMMUS

Yield: 3-4 servings

Ingredients

1 can chickpeas, rinsed and drained
1 can black beans, rinsed and drained
1/3 cup tahini (sesame seed paste)
¼ cup extra-virgin olive oil
1 clove garlic, minced (use 2 if they're small)
1 teaspoon ground cumin
1 teaspoon low sodium salt
3 tablespoons fresh lemon or lime juice
Cayenne pepper, to taste

Directions

1. In a blender, combine all the ingredients and pulse until smooth. You can add a little olive oil or water if it is too thick.
2. You can adjust the seasoning by adding more lemon or lime juice, salt and cayenne.
3. Serve.

Drinks Recipes

A MESSAGE FOR READERS

The recipes listed under Drinks section are extremely healthy and nutritious for Gout. You may or can adjust the quantity of ingredients based on the servings you are preparing.

CUCUMBER & GINGER DRINK

Yield: 1 serving

Ingredients

1 medium-sized cucumber
2 ribs of celery
A slice of lemon
1-inch young ginger root

Directions

1. Start by cleaning the ingredients thoroughly.
2. Next step is to cut the cucumber into smaller pieces.
3. Prepare the celery ribs by making sure that there is no dirt on them.
4. Cut the lemon into half.
5. Then carve out the ginger root.
6. Juice all in a juicer.

PINEAPPLE, TURMERIC, GINGER & CHERRY DRINK

Yield: 1 serving

Ingredients

1 pineapple
1-2 teaspoons of powdered turmeric
2-3 teaspoons of powdered ginger, or 1 inch off of a fresh ginger root
1 cup of tart cherry juice

Directions

1. Start by cutting the skin and removing the stem of the pineapple. Slice the pineapple into small chunks of quite same size. Toss the chunks in a blender or food processor.
2. Whirl the pineapple chunks until they are mashed up evenly. Now, pour 1 cup of tart cherry juice and sprinkle 2-3 teaspoons of ginger powder and 1 to 2 teaspoons of turmeric.
3. Blend well. Serve.
4. You can store this drink in an airtight glass container in the refrigerator for up to a week and a half.

GOUT PAIN RELIEVING DRINK
COMBO 1

Yield: 1 serving

Ingredients

2 green apples
2 ribs celery
1 small or ½, a large cucumber
¼ bitter gourd, small (optional as it is bitter)
¼ lemon
Thumb-sized ginger

Directions

1. Start by cleaning and washing all the ingredients thoroughly.
2. Juice all the ingredients in the juicer and serve.

GOUT PAIN RELIEVING DRINK COMBO 2

Yield: 1 serving

Ingredients

2 carrots
1 cucumber
8 ribs of celery

Directions

1. Start by cleaning and washing all the ingredients thoroughly.
2. Juice all the ingredients in the juicer and serve.

GOUT PAIN RELIEVING DRINK

COMBO 3

Yield: 1 serving

Ingredients

2 green apples
1 cucumber
1 fennel
6 leaves of big kale
¼ lemon slice
Thumb-size ginger

Directions

1. Start by cleaning and washing all the ingredients thoroughly.
2. Juice all the ingredients in the juicer and serve.

GOUT PAIN RELIEVING DRINK
COMBO 4

Yield: 1 serving

Ingredients

2 green apples (or chayote)
6 ribs of celery
¼ cabbage
Thumb-size ginger

Directions

1. Start by cleaning and washing all the ingredients thoroughly.
2. Juice all the ingredients in the juicer and serve.

GOUT PAIN RELIEVING DRINK

COMBO 5

Yield: 1 serving

Ingredients

2 carrots
½ celeriac
1 fennel
1 cucumber
¼ lemon slice

Directions

1. Start by cleaning and washing all the ingredients thoroughly.
2. Juice all the ingredients in the juicer and serve.

GOUT PAIN RELIEVING DRINK

COMBO 6

Yield: 1 serving

Ingredients

1 green apples
1 cucumber
1 small bitter gourd
¼ lemon slice

Directions

1. Start by cleaning and washing all the ingredients thoroughly.
2. Juice all the ingredients in the juicer and serve.

GOUT PAIN RELIEVING DRINK
COMBO 7

Yield: 1 serving

Ingredients

1 cucumber
1 medium-sized beetroot
¼ lemon slice
Thumb-size ginger

Directions

1. Start by cleaning and washing all the ingredients thoroughly.
2. Juice all the ingredients in the juicer and serve.

GOUT PAIN RELIEVING DRINK

COMBO 8

Yield: 1 serving

Ingredients

6 ribs of celery
½ small pineapple
¼ lemon
Thumb-size ginger

Directions

1. Start by cleaning and washing all the ingredients thoroughly.
2. Juice all the ingredients in the juicer and serve.

Desserts Recipes

A MESSAGE FOR READERS

The recipes listed under Desserts section are extremely healthy and nutritious for Gout. You may or can adjust the quantity of ingredients based on the servings you are preparing.

MANGO & RICE PUDDING

Yield: 2-4 servings

Ingredients

1 ripe mango, peeled and cubed
1 cup jasmine rice, drained
3 cups low-fat milk
½ cup low-fat coconut milk

Directions

1. Take a heavy saucepan and combine all the ingredients.
2. Bring it to a boil. Let it cook for about 30 minutes on a low heat.
3. Once cooked, remove from the heat. Pour the pudding into dessert bowls.
4. Cool and serve.

CHOCOLATY STRAWBERRIES

Yield: 4-5 servings

Ingredients

1½ pounds fresh strawberries
10 oz. dark chocolate (at least 60% cocoa content), melted
½ cup coconut flakes
¼ cup almond slices

Directions

1. Prepare a baking sheet by placing a baking paper on it. Set aside.
2. Now, dip the strawberries one by one into the melted chocolate. Then roll the strawberries either through almonds or coconut flakes.
3. Place them onto the baking sheet.
4. Refrigerate them for about 10 minutes to allow the chocolate to set.
5. Serve.

SUGAR FREE CHOCO MOUSSE

Yield: 2-4 servings

Ingredients

1 ripe avocado, peeled
1 ripe banana
1 teaspoon lemon juice
¼ cup dark cocoa powder
2 oz. dark chocolate (at least 60% cocoa content), melted

Directions

1. In a blender, combine all the ingredients.
2. Now, pulse until smooth and well blended.
3. Use a spoon to transfer the mousse to individual dessert bowls.
4. Serve immediately.

SIMPLY BAKED PEARS

Yield: 4 servings

Ingredients

4 pears
Honey
Cinnamon
Low-fat butter

Directions

1. Start by slicing the pears into half and the laying them on a baking sheet. Please make sure to scoop the seeds out.
2. Rub each half of the pear with cinnamon, honey and low-fat butter.
3. Finally, bake at 350 degrees F for about 30 to 45 minutes. Pears will be pretty soft when done.
4. Serve.

DELICIOUS RICE PUDDING

Yield: 12 servings

Ingredients

1 cup uncooked white rice = 3 cups cooked white rice
3 cups low-fat milk
2 tbsp. low-fat margarine
½ cup sugar substitute
½ cup raisins
1 tsp. vanilla extract
½ tsp. nutmeg
1 tsp. cinnamon

Directions

1. First step is to cook the rice. To cook the rice, use 1 cup dry white rice and 2 cups of water. Once cooked, let the rice cool down for few minutes.
2. Take a medium sized pot and mix the milk, rice, sugar substitute, raisins, margarine and vanilla. Now, cook for about 25 minutes over medium heat or until the liquid is pretty much absorbed. Stir frequently in between.
3. Now, add the nutmeg and cinnamon. Stir well.
4. Let it cook for another 5 minutes.
5. Serve either hot or cold.

PART C - THE PREVENTION AND CURE GUIDE

This Page Has Been Left Blank Intentionally.

Chapter 9

The Prevention of Gout

Do not think of gout as an old fashioned disease that it is known to be. Regardless of what others say, it is a big deal! Gout is way more widespread than it should be and can cause a lot of pain and discomfort when left untreated. There are many ways to process uric acids in your blood streams and diet has to be one of the most crucial ways to prevent gout. Even maintaining healthy weight in addition to taking medications may also help you in preventing this pervasive disease.

Here are some tips that you can use to prevent gout in the first place.

Aim for a Healthy Body Weight

Sometimes when you are overweight and you take the crash diet route, you become exposed to more damage than good. Your body weight plays a huge role in preventing or exacerbating the gout. Don't just willy-nilly jump onto new diets. Always rope in your doctor and avoid restrictive diet.

If you must lose weight, it should be done slowly and steadily. If you are already a candidate of gout, dropping pounds too quickly can actually trigger an attack by stressing your kidney's ability to process harmful ingredients. High-protein, starvation or diets rich in diuretic supplements are harmful for people who are at risk of gout.

Follow a Routine of Exercise

When you want to lose weight, any physical activity will be helpful and will contribute towards healthy weight loss. You can also reduce the risk associated with gout when you make a routine of exercising daily. You don't have to do anything heavy duty. Just moderate activity such as cycling, brisk walking, swimming or running for at least 2.5 hours every week should do the trick.

Take Help from a Professional

If you are bringing in diet changes and have not been able to notice any progress towards healthy weight loss, you must consult a medically trained expert for supervision. Since gout can be triggered for so many reasons, it is better to take your consultation from someone who is an expert on the subject.

Ask for Medication If Lifestyle Changes Are Not Enough

If you notice that a healthy lifestyle and dietary guidelines are not helping, you can also take medication that your doctor prescribes. Follow the instructions to the rote as taking too much medication can also have its own ill effects, making the gout even worse than before.

Check for Poisoning By Lead

According to a recent research, one more factor that can cause gout is the lead poisoning, even if the levels of uric acid are low. Even though there are more studies required to confirm this fact, you can still check with your doctor to test your blood or hair for toxins. If you have been living in a building that uses lead based paint regularly or work in an industrial area, then it would be a good idea to get yourself checked for lead poisoning.

Avoid Diuretic Medication

These medications are used as dietary supplements and may possibly worsen the gout condition. Ask your doctor if you are administered any medicines that contain diuretics and if you can take potassium supplement to counter its affect.

This Page Has Been Left Blank Intentionally.

Chapter 10

The Natural Medications –
Benefits & Side Effects

Gout can be very painful and in that moment you will look for anything to just make the pain go away and gain back your mobility. This is also the time when you feel inclined to give natural medication a shot. However, the question is, are these medications a good substitute, or even a viable addition to your existing treatment?

The people who promote natural cures and healing believe otherwise. According to them, all these advertisements about medicines treating your gout are just pharmaceutical companies wearing a garb of your trusted doctor. They say that your doctor perhaps doesn't even know how to treat gout in addition to your other problems. Is it true? Are the newfangled "natural" medicines really challenging the whole foundation of medical treatment of gout?

The people who did not benefit much from their regular medicines may fall for this perspective. It is easy to call your doctors "misinformed" about the condition and its treatment. However, just think about it, if you have a hard time trusting your GP, what makes you believe in this anonymous "natural medicines" website that "assures" results? How do you know there aren't any serious side effects of this medication? Who is to say that it is really an alternative or additional treatment for your gout?

Here, we share some natural medicines that are said to treat gout, albeit with its own set of side effects. Be informed before you make a choice.

Natural Medicines and their Side Effects

Before you pounce at the organic medicines, it is important for you to know that these drugs are made from highly concentrated forms of herbal extracts and are not regulated by the FDA. Hence, there is no trusted authority that can prove its efficacy. The one thing you must note is that all these medicines are quite obviously very expensive and almost guarantee that there are no side effects. But is it really true?

Like we said before, these medicines are highly concentrated forms of pharmaceutical drugs. The substance that does supposedly help you is not added in a controlled amount; instead the entire extract is used. There is also a possibility that even though you are taking the herb that does treat gout, your medicines do not have enough dosage to make the impact.

So before you choose the natural treatment, let us discuss some natural treatments and their side effects.

Saponins or Yucca Stalk

Yucca is known for its inherent properties in metabolizing purine, the leading cause of gout. It was used by the Native Americans for hundreds of years as an indigenous treatment of gout. However, this herb can cause diarrhea. If used for a long time, it can also affect the absorption of fat soluble vitamins such as Vitamins A, D, E and K.

Milk Thistle

This herb, also known as silymarin, is responsible for liver production and also stimulates new liver cell growth. When in your body, it can help boost the aspirin effects and protect you from potential overdose if your liver is damaged. It is also used in chemotherapies and is beneficial in type II diabetes. You can choose to consume milk thistle if you have complaints such as Cirrhosis, hepatitis or any other inflammatory liver condition.

Milk Thistle may be a Mediterranean native but it is being grown all around the world because of its medicinal properties. They are easily identifiable as plants with a long stem, and leaves around 4-10 feet wide that are marked with white veins. The silymarin found in milk thistle is the main substance that is known to protect the liver cells. It does so in three ways:

- Helps cells from damage during body's oxidation process due to its antioxidant properties
- Liver cells are protected against swelling up due to its anti-inflammatory properties
- Promotes liver cell growth and stops toxins from entering the liver cells.

The recent research proves that milk thistle helps your liver and protects it against conditions such as cirrhosis, hepatitis and other inflammatory conditions. Scientists also believe that it can also protect the body against skin cancer, allergies and high cholesterol. It is the antioxidant property of the herb that has incredible healing power, say scientists. It is also believed that milk thistle allows the body to discharge toxins more quickly. Its extracts are examined as a way to decrease the liver damage of a person who is undergoing chemotherapy.

- ## Dosage

Milk thistle is available in many different forms such as soft gels, tinctures, tablets and capsules. To mitigate the liver problem, you will be required to take between 400 and 600 mg everyday broken into three equal doses. It is advised to consult your doctor before you take the milk thistle so that you can ensure that it is not interfering with any other medication that you might be taking.

- ## Side effects

The problem with toxins and their exit from the body is that they often put up a strong fight before they are extricated. Don't be surprised if you experience bloating, feel full, changes in bowel habits, diarrhea, headache, rhino-conjunctivitis and even anaphylaxis in some cases.

Milk thistle is readily available in health stores. However, before you pick up a bottle off the aisle, make sure that you read the label carefully so that you are getting home the purest form of the extracts and not something mixed with chemicals.

Sativum or Ripened Garlic

You can take aged garlic to detoxify your body with no significant side effects. The only flip side to using this herb is bad breath. However, the best way to consume sativum is by adding it to your diet, without actually paying for it. The high sulfur content in aged garlic is very good for overall health and well-being.

Turmeric

The anti-inflammatory properties of turmeric are well known and so is its potency for liver protection. Turmeric is used extensively in Indian cuisines and helps the cancer patients who undergo chemotherapy. However, it is important to note that turmeric may cause gallstones, as per some studies.

Artichoke Powder

Powdered form of artichoke leads to bile production. Even though there are no known side effects, you can simply add artichokes to your salad and enjoy the same benefits as its powdered form. It is not really required to buy it as a supplement.

There are many other herbs that may be effective for the treatment of the gout but their side effects are something that will never be revealed by the cure seller. It is also possible that they tell you not to use the prescription drugs at all and make their cure the ultimate solution to the problem. Rather than falling for it, use your own research and consult professionals before you take such a drastic step. If you really must reap the benefits of these herbs, you can also explore the possibility of adding them to your diet rather than paying a fortune for their extracts.

This Page Has Been Left Blank Intentionally.

Chapter 11

Managing Gout – No Magic, Just Simple Solution

There are many people that are often disturbed by the untimely gout flare ups and the way it impacts their lives. However, the good news is that there is a solution and a very simple one at that! Many people may not know that but managing gout is no rocket science, it is actually quite uncomplicated.

We just discussed how herbs may be an alternative solution to your problem and the best herbs to tackle gout flare-ups is celery seed and devil's claw. Let us discuss each individually and learn why they are important.

Celery Seed

Celery seeds are popular not just because they give us the celery we eat in our soups and salads but it is also recognized as a strong medicinal herb. These therapeutic seeds are extracted from the flowered plant. The celery seeds have a history of medicinal remedy in several parts of the world. As the plant reaches its second year, the celery seeds are harvested. Their seeds and stalk are a powerhouse of compounds such as vitamins A, C, E and K, iron, minerals, magnesium, calcium, amino acids, and essential oils. Celery seeds are known to be very useful for the treatment of conditions such as indigestion, gout and arthritis.

History of Celery Seeds

Celery has been used by the ancient Egyptians as food and even its leaves were found in King Tutankhamen's tomb. Ancient Rome and Greece also used its seeds for medicinal purposes and food. In 30 AD, the Roman King Aulus Cornelius Celcus learned that celery is effective against pain and inflammation. The herbalist from Europe, Nicholas Culpeper wrote in a paper in 1653 that celery can purify your blood and make it sweet.

Celery Seed's role in Gout Relief

It is the diuretic properties of celery seeds that make it so valuable for gout treatment. It aids fluid retention and also cleanses the body of needle-like uric acid crystals that are the main cause of gout and its flare up. The antiseptic properties of celery seeds also help treat the urinary tract inflammation. Celery seeds also help in building overall healthy body and can be used interchangeably with the medication allopurinol, a medicine that helps the body get rid of excess uric acid. 2-4 tablets of celery seed extract every day may be sufficient in preventing the gout attack.

Precautions

Since celery seeds may cause photosensitivity, its use should be avoided in the sun. Pregnant women are also cautioned against using the celery seed extracts. People with kidney disease should use these extract in supervision of their doctors. It is recommended to eat high potassium foods when you are taking celery seed extracts as it is a strong diuretic and can exhaust your body's supply.

The most common side effect of celery seeds is diarrhea. Stop taking celery seeds if you experience an upset stomach.

Quick treatment for Gout Flare-up

Use one teaspoon of crushed celery seeds to make a cup of tea. Just add it to the boiling water and let it steep for 10-15 minutes before straining into a cup. Drink this tea up to three times a day to treat gout pains.

Devils Claw

Devil's claw is apparently one of the most effective remedies associated with the symptoms and pains related to gout. Also, known as wood spider and grapple plant, Devil's Claw is a South African native where it has been used for over a thousand years as a medicinal herb. While the whole plant comes packed with rich healing benefits, it is the root that has the power to reduce fever, treat stomach problems and also fix the symptoms of arthritis.

Replenishing your Nutrients Reserve

Devil's Claw helps adding the nutrients back into the body. This herb includes minerals such as iron, calcium, magnesium, manganese and also sodium, selenium and silicon. It also stocks up your protein reserve while adding crucial vitamins A and C into your diet. An addition to its numerous benefits, it is also an excellent cleanser that removes toxins and impurities from your body making you feel healthier than ever!

Natural Remedy for Gout

The nutritional benefit notwithstanding, the Devil's claw is known for its characteristic iridoids, the main component that has powerful anti-inflammatory properties. If you suffer from gout, you will be able to see why this herb is a powerful solution for the condition. Not only will your joint inflammation will be relieved significantly, it also acts as a vital pain reliever.

The improper digestion of protein plays an active role in flaring up gout. The Devil's claw works as a digestive stimulant and can prove to be helpful. It is the combination of these two properties that makes Devil's Claw such a popular choice for treating this health problem. Many people will be happy to vouch for the positive impact of this herb on their condition.

How to Use Devil's Claw?

There are many ways to use the herb. However, be sure to read the instructions on the label for its safe usage. No matter in what form you are taking the herb, just tweak the dosage accordingly. It is also possible to consume it in tea form. Another popular form of Devil's Claw is the lotion or cream that you can apply to the affected areas. However, regardless of how you use it, it is always better to consume it in a single format or you can risk overdose.

Precautions

Some things must be taken into consideration when you consume Devil's Claw. Despite its effectiveness, it is advised to prevent its use unless you have your doctor's supervision. It is also better to refrain from using this herb if you have diabetes, blood pressure or recurrent stomach problems. Only buy your medication from a reputable source so that you can get the best quality product. Pregnant women are advised against its use.

This Page Has Been Left Blank Intentionally.

Chapter 12

The Oil Treatment for Gout

Another way to treat the inflammation caused by gout is to use topical application of oil. Here are some popular options you can consider to allay your condition.

Arnica

Arnica is such a valuable herb that it has been used in pretty much all the branches of medicine – allopathic, herbal, homeopathic, you name it! Arnica has been a part of American and European science for centuries. Both the cultures used Arnica and forms of it for treating pains and curing bruises and also fixing the wounds.

The plant of Arnica is perineal and has flowers that look like daisies. According to the researchers, the herb contains helenalin and dihydrohelenalin that contain analgesic and anti-inflammatory properties. Even though Arnica is very efficient when used topically on wounds, its ingestion can just as easily become toxic. It is also known to affect the heart and the circulatory system adversely. Several times helenalin can cause allergic reaction on your skin.

Benefits

Arnica is popularly used as an ointment for bruises, aches, wounds, swelling from fracture, rheumatism, and insect bite inflammation. It is also used in homeopathy treatments for mitigating muscle soreness, and alleviating conditions like trauma and anxiety. Since homeopathy preparations use very small quantity of plant molecules, they are considered absolutely safe for use if taken under your doctor's guidance.

Epsom Salts

There are many ways in which Epsom salts can be beneficial for you. The salts are made of Magnesium and Sulfates that can help you ease the stress and also improve your concentration, thus positively impacting your sleep cycles. However, the core benefit of Epsom Salts with reference to gout is that by adding just a few teaspoons to your bath water, you can actually treat your muscle soreness and joint inflammation. The magnesium present in the salts is an electrolyte that can help you make sure that your muscles function properly. It is also crucial for the way calcium is absorbed and utilized by your body. Even though there is magnesium present in your food, the best way to take it in is through absorption.

It is the way it regulates the 325+ enzymes in your body that works its magic in relieving pain and muscle cramps. Your body's insulin becomes more effective, helping the body to perform with the right sugar levels. The bottom line is that magnesium directs the way your body uses oxygen.

The second component, Sulfates, found in Epsom Salts also help you remove toxins and positively impact the way your body absorbs nutrients. It is also very crucial in brain development and its role with joint proteins.

There are many ways to use Epsom salts. Just add 2 cups of salt per gallon of water and use it for treatment of muscle soreness, splinter removal and bug bites. You can also use it in a soaking bath.

Cayenne Pepper

Grown in several parts of the world, Cayenne pepper was first used in Latin America as a seasoning spice. However, with time it was realized that it is not only flavorful but also healthy because it holds many healing properties.

For centuries, Cayenne pepper has been used to treat bloating, cramps, stomach pains, gastrointestinal problems and also the circulatory troubles. It was first introduced by Christopher Columbus to Europe after he discovered the Caribbean Islands.

The Magical Healing Properties

The most well-known healing potential of Cayenne pepper is its ability to treat the gastrointestinal tract. Cayenne not only soothes indigestion but when used externally, it can also be helpful with pain associated with rheumatism and arthritis. The active component, capsaicin, found in Cayenne peppers is helpful in treating fibromyalgia after being made into a lotion that is massaged onto joints and muscles that hurt. It is the capsaicin present in the pepper that is effective for treatment of pain and discomfort. It is not only an effective solution to treat body's discomfort; it is also a very good antioxidant.

Blood Sugar levels

One more essential benefit of cayenne pepper is to bring down the blood sugar levels naturally for someone who is diabetic. All it takes is a moderate dose of capsaicin to bring down the high blood sugar levels.

Arthritis

When consumed regularly, cayenne pepper can block the Nerve Growth Factor. As a result, a hormone called Substance P is stimulated that sends pain signals from the body to the brain. When this hormone is blocked, at first a large amount of substance P is released by the body that can increase the pain substantially but then it diminishes, thus relieving the arthritic pain.

The people who are suffering from arthritis, the signs of improvement can be seen when there is no feeling of pain. Cayenne can also boost the endorphins production, which are the natural painkillers produced by the body. When you take the Cayenne pepper dosage of 2-3 capsules every day, pain will initially increase and then eventually exit from the body leaving the person pain free!

Side Effects

Apart from the burning sensation felt after using Cayenne pepper, there are also minor side effects. Never touch sensitive areas such as your eyes after handling the pepper. Also note that after ingesting it for too long, you may also experience ulcers.

This Page Has Been Left Blank Intentionally.

Chapter 13

The Body Therapies for Gout

There are many complementary therapies that help relieve gout with absolutely no side effects. In fact, when used over a period of time, it can also unleash several health benefits of its own. Let us discuss some more therapies that you can consider alongside your gout treatment.

Aromatherapy

The gout arthritis is so painful and disruptive that you are willing to try every new therapy on the block! All you want to do is cure your common problems and start feeling better. One of the most well-known methods to alleviate your painful gout is the aromatherapy session.

The aromatherapy, as the name suggests, uses scents as the major part of its therapy. There are many different kinds of scents that can be used for your healing, depending upon your preference and your condition. The scents are either used in bath or through a massage. You can also inhale them directly. However, it is the application of scents that determine what it is being used for. For instance, if you want a treatment for your arthritis then you need to get a massage therapy.

For the treatment to be effective, it is imperative that the scents used in aromatherapy are completely environmental. These scents are obtained naturally from the plants, flowers, trees, and other components found in the nature. It is important to remember that the artificial scents don't really work in aromatherapy sessions. This is why you should use absolutely authentic oils/scents for your treatment.

It doesn't matter what is the purpose of your therapy, it may be used for treating your gout or heal any other condition, but aromatherapy is a tried and tested method that has proved its potency in science and personal experience.

Hydrotherapy

It is so annoying when your feet swell up and your entire body hurts. All you want is to get relief from gout and you have tried all the methods there are. However, there is one more thing you can try before you give up all hope, hydrotherapy.

While keeping yourself hydrated is a magic mantra to relieve not one but many ailments, preventing gout is now another thing you can add to the list. Hydrotherapy uses the combination of hot and cold water to treat gout externally and is a great method to relieve pain that comes from your gout. By drinking plenty of water throughout the day, you can keep your joints lubricated which prevent the outbreak of attacks. When combined with hydrotherapy, the benefits and relief from gout will come sooner than you expected. There are two ways to use hydrotherapy for gout; Contrast and Standard.

Contrast Hydrotherapy

To dissolve urate crystals in your joints during gout attack by using the hot and cold compresses technique is called the Contrast method. This method also helps reduce pain and inflammation in the area. The compresses are altered between hot one being used for three minutes then switched with cold one for thirty seconds. No more than 20 minutes should be spent on the therapy and it should be ended with a cold compress.

Standard Hydrotherapy

In this therapy, the body is submerged in hot water. The bubbling jets in your bathtub can dilate the blood vessels that improve the blood circulation and the flow of oxygen is increased in the body. This process releases natural pain killers throughout your body. Sore joints experience instant relief through this method. The only word of caution is to take your doctor's advice before starting hydrotherapy.

Reflexology

Reflexology is also one of the most commonly known methods to treat gout effectively. It is also called zone therapy and is used not in conjunction but as an alternative to using pills and/or injections to mitigate the pain. This therapy involves stimulating specific points on your hands, ears and feet that double up as pressure points. This therapy is very effective and promotes positive healing. Although this treatment can improve overall health, but for the treatment of gout it is administered to the feet so that pain can be relieved for the person suffering from this symptom.

Reflexology is not a scientific procedure but uses a qualified practitioner to apply the correct pressure on areas of bare feet while massaging it with hands. After massage, the blood circulation in the body improves that also helps in removing toxins and increasing the absorption of nutrients and oxygen in body cells. As a result, your body becomes better capable of managing pain and dealing with stress.

Using reflexology on someone suffering from gout will aid in restoring the kidney's balance. Since it is the kidneys that are responsible for the production of uric acid, the benefit of this treatment is understandable. By stimulating the feet, the body's energy aligns with the kidneys that can help lower the production of uric acid. It is also a beneficial method for breaking the uric acids crystal deposits that contribute to gout pain in the big toe region.

Even though this treatment does not have any side-effects, some people do experience nausea, sinus and congestion that is caused by body's release of toxins. The symptoms do not last more than 24 hours.

Acupuncture Treatment

Acupuncture originates from the ancient Chinese practice that has been traced back to the Stone Age. You may or may not believe in the effectiveness of the treatment but the concept is logical and is based on the belief that our body contains 14 channels that carry energy and by stimulating these channels any pain can be relieved, even if it is gout.

The points in the body are rubbed with alcohol and then a very thin needle is inserted into each point. There are many points where the needles can be inserted at different depths where they can stay inside from a few minutes to an hour. When in the process of the treatment, the needles are gently spun so as to energize the region electrically. When your body becomes charged, you may feel a sense of tingling underneath your skin. Soon you will feel the pain waning off from your body.

Acupressure

Acupressure can be a great alternative to modern medicine. It is more a therapy than a medical process. According to researchers, it can be an effective method in prevention and treatment of many diseases. It is also being actively used to relieve the symptoms of gout.

Acupressure is relatively less heard of than its ancient Chinese cousin, Acupuncture. In principle, both the therapies are quite similar. However, the only difference is that while acupuncture is performed with needles, acupressure uses hands and feet to apply pressure to different points on the body. This technique is built on body's natural ability to self-heal. The blood circulation is increased by stimulating the body using pressure. The muscular tension can be felt dissipating as the pressure is gently applied to the skin's surface using hand, knuckles and even feet sometimes. This is a great method for someone who is suffering from gout to release some of the pain caused by inflammation.

How does it work?

The body has 2,000 areas that are activated as the energy passes throughout the body. This energy is called Chi or Qi and is said to flow from the skin's surface into the body's internal organs. These paths of energy flow are called meridians. There are about 20 meridians in our body and if there is illness or injury, these meridians get blocked and the flow of energy is also disrupted. This energy flow is unblocked using the acupressure which allows the mind and body to attain the natural state of balance.

People that are suffering from joint pain or inflammation can experience pain at anytime, anywhere. This is why they often feel hard to relax. Acupressure can treat these symptoms and a lot more by simply applying appropriate pressure to specific points on the surface of the body. As a result, the blood flow increases and the muscles start to relax.

There are many ways in which gout sufferers are able to gain respite through acupressure technique, such as:

- Release of tension from the body
- Improved blood circulation
- Pain relief
- Reduction in stress
- Relief in inflamed areas
- Clarity of mind

How does it help?

While anyone can learn to apply pressure to their trigger points, it is recommended to take help from the professional first and learn the proper technique. The doctor applies pressure on each trigger point for about 30 seconds. At first, one would feel a jolt in the area and then the spot will be stimulated. However, over a period of time, the treatment's sensitivity decreases. You can use acupressure therapy in addition to your medication for best results. Do consult your doctor before undergoing any remedy, even if it is acupressure.

Meditation

Meditation is one of those methods that not only eases gout symptoms but also improves your overall health. Through meditation, you would be able to clear your mind, eliminate stress and increase your body's efficiency. People who practice this ancient art of holistic healing say that through meditation, one can experience an instant effect on their physical as well as mental state. All you need is to learn how to channel your thoughts in a single space and then concentrate. You can start by sitting in a quite spot and center all your focus on a light or a sound to train your brain.

The way your body can align our breath to our mind is where the trick of meditation lies. When you meditate, the focus on your breathing can bring your mind and body together. This process works wonders in decreasing the stress hormone, cortisol, and also decreases the heart rate and blood pressure.

Studies even prove that by meditating, you can improve your body's ability to tolerate pain, increase activity levels, self-esteem and reduce stress, anxiety, depression and sometime later, even medication. Many patients have reported success by using the mindfulness meditation that helps in relieving pain, enhancing mood in patients suffering from chronic pain, including chest pain, low back pain, headache and gastrointestinal pain.

Since the number of people suffering from gout and arthritis pain have increased significantly, the use of yoga and meditation have emerged as top practices along with medication to help promote overall well-being. Meditation has been proven to help the sufferers of arthritis by decreasing pain in the inflamed joints by taking their mind off their suffering.

Even insomnia can be treated with meditation. You may often feel sleepless, if your eating habits are bad, you are living a stressful life or do not exercise enough. Your biorhythms get affected due to decreased melatonin levels, which lead to insomnia. The feel good hormone, melatonin, increases when one meditates regularly.

You can also take your mind off your condition and realign your focus in life's positive aspects. This reduces the stress and enhances your mood. As your muscles relax, your blood pressure returns to normal and your heart beats at a standard pace. You start to feel better as your body releases endorphins. If you need a healthy and a cost-effective method, you can certainly look at meditation as an important part of your wellness plan.

Wrapping up!

According to another study, as many as 78% doctors don't know how to treat gout properly. In this case, it is guides like these that can help you understand your condition so that you can empower yourself with knowledge and align your treatment with the symptoms by educating yourself.

At last, I would like to thank you for reading this book and hope that you will create a new healthier you!

This Page Has Been Left Blank Intentionally.

RECIPES INDEX

29022765R00109

Made in the USA
Lexington, KY
24 January 2019